Basic Medical Terminology

Concise Memorization and Comprehension Course

Subcourse MD0010

Edition 100

AF873728

Basic Medical Terminology

Concise Memorization and Comprehension Course

Subcourse MD0010

Edition 100

Basic Medical Terminology: Concise Memorization and Comprehension Course
Subcourse MD0010

PharmaLogika

PharmaLogika, Inc.
PO Box 461
Willow Springs, NC 27592

www.pharmalogika.com

PharmaLogika Books is an imprint of PharmaLogika, Inc. PharmaLogika and its logos are trademarks of PharmaLogika, Inc. All other trademarks used herein are the properties of their respective owners and are used for identification purposes only.

Author / Editor: Mindy J. Allport-Settle

Published by PharmaLogika, Inc.

Printed in the United States of America.

ISBN 0-9830719-8-5
ISBN-13 978-0-9830719-8-3

Contents

Overview

About this Book

The United States Army is recognized internationally as the standard for complete, efficient and effective adult education. The Army has a tradition of pioneering training systems (including computer-based training) that then transition into the corporate sector. This manual has been continuously tested and updated to successfully educate every member of the modern United States Army. The needs of the instructor, the student, and the Army are perfectly balanced. This is the model all educators strive to follow when developing and delivering training programs.

Included Documents and Features

Basic Medical Terminology

1. Introduction to Programmed Learning
2. Stems Pertaining to Medical Terminology
3. Prefixes Pertaining to Medical Terminology
4. Suffixes Pertaining to Medical Terminology

- Pre-tests and Self Assessments for each Lesson
- Complete Glossary
- Pronunciation Guide
- Abbreviations and Symbols
- Final Examination

Orientation

Medical Terminology

Medical terminology is the vocabulary and structure of words used to accurately describe the human body and associated components, conditions, and processes in a concise and scientific manner. This systematic approach to word building and term comprehension is based on the concept of: (1) word roots, (2) prefixes, and (3) suffixes. The word root is a term derived from a source language such as Greek or Latin and usually describes a part of the body. The prefix can be added in front of the term to modify the word root by giving additional information about the location of an organ, the number of parts, or time involved. Suffixes are attached to the end of a word root to add meaning such as condition, disease process, or procedure.

In the process of creating medical terminology, certain rules of language apply. These rules are part of language mechanics called linguistics. Medical terminology also follows a logical process of word construction so that even an unfamiliar term can be identified.

Army Medical Command

The U.S. Army Medical Command (MEDCOM) is a major command of the U.S. Army that provides command and control of the Army's fixed-facility medical, dental, and veterinary treatment facilities, providing preventive care, medical research and development and training institutions.

Structure and Subordinate Commands

MEDCOM is divided into Regional Medical Commands that oversee day-to-day operations in military treatment facilities, exercising command and control over the medical treatment facilities in their regions. There are currently five of these regional commands:

- Europe Regional Medical Command
- Southern Regional Medical Command
- Northern Regional Medical Command

- Pacific Regional Medical Command
- Western Regional Medical Command.

Additional subordinate commands of MEDCOM include:

- Army Medical Department Center & School (AMEDDC&S)
- U.S. Army Public Health Command (Provisional), (known as the U.S. Army Center for Health Promotion & Preventive Medicine prior to 1 October 2009 {USACHPPM or CHPPM})
- U.S. Army Medical Research and Materiel Command (USAMRMC)
- Warrior Transition Command (WTC)
- U.S. Army Dental Command (DENCOM)

Operations

In Garrison (Peacetime)

MEDCOM maintains day-to-day health care for soldiers, retired soldiers and the families of both. Despite the wide range of responsibilities involved in providing health care in traditional settings as well as on the battlefield, the Army Medical Department's quality of care compares very favorably with that of civilian health organizations, when measured by civilian standards. Many Army medical facilities report on their own quality-of-care standards on their individual Internet sites.

Deployments

When Army field hospitals deploy, most clinical professional and support personnel come from MEDCOM's fixed facilities. In addition to support of combat operations, deployments can be for humanitarian assistance, peacekeeping, and other stability and support operations. Under the Professional Officer Filler System (PROFIS), up to 26 percent of MEDCOM physicians and 43 percent of MEDCOM nurses are sent to field units during a full deployment. To replace PROFIS losses, Reserve units and Individual Mobilization Augmentees (non-unit reservists) are mobilized to work in medical treatment facilities. The department also provides trained medical specialists to the Army's combat medical units, which are assigned directly to combatant commanders.

Many Army Reserve and Army National Guard units deploy in support of the Army Medical Department. The Army depends heavily on its Reserve component for medical support—about 63 percent of the Army's medical forces are in the Reserve component.

Army Medical Department

The Army Medical Department of the U.S. Army (AMEDD) comprises the Army's six medical Special Branches (or "Corps") of officers and medical enlisted soldiers. It was established as the "Army Hospital" in July 1775 to coordinate the medical care required by the Continental Army during the Revolutionary War. The AMEDD is led by the Surgeon General of the U.S. Army, a lieutenant general.

The AMEDD is the U.S. Army's healthcare organization, not a U.S. Army command. The AMEDD is found in all three components of the Army: the Active Army, the U.S. Army Reserve, and the Army National Guard. Its headquarters are at Fort Sam Houston, San Antonio, Texas, which hosts the AMEDD Center and School. Equal numbers of AMEDD senior leaders can be found in Washington D.C., divided between the Pentagon and the Walter Reed Army Medical Center (WRAMC).

The Academy of Health Sciences, under the Army Medical Department Center & School, provides training to the officers and enlisted soldiers of the AMEDD. As a result of BRAC 2005, enlisted medical training was transferred to the new Medical Education and Training Campus, consolidating most military enlisted medical training at Fort Sam Houston.[1]

Medical Special Branches

- Medical Corps (MC)
- Nurse Corps (AN)
- Dental Corps (DC)
- Veterinary Corps (VC)
- Medical Service Corps (MS)

[1] U.S. Army Medical Department AMEDD Center and School Portal available on the Internet at: http://www.cs.amedd.army.mil/. Additional information specific to the Fort Sam Houston consolidation is available n the Internet at: http://www.aetc.af.mil/shared/media/document/AFD-071026-035.pdf

- Medical Specialist Corps (AMSC)

United States Army Training and Doctrine Command

Established 1 July 1973, the United States Army Training and Doctrine Command (TRADOC) is an army command of the United States Army headquartered at Fort Monroe, Virginia. It is charged with overseeing training of Army forces, the development of operational doctrine, and the development and procurement of new weapons systems. TRADOC operates 33 schools and centers at 16 Army installations. TRADOC schools conduct 2,734 courses (81 directly in support of mobilization) and 373 language courses. The 2,734 courses include 503,164 seats for 434,424 soldiers; 34,675 other-service personnel; 7,824 international soldiers; and 26,241 civilians.[2]

TRADOC MissionThe official mission statement for TRADOC states:

> TRADOC develops the Army's Soldiers and Civilian leaders and designs, develops and integrates capabilities, concepts and doctrine in order to build a campaign-capable, expeditionary Army in support of joint warfighting capability through Army Force Generation (ARFORGEN).[3]

TRADOC is the official command component that is responsible for training and developing the United States Army.

TRADOC History

TRADOC was established as a major U.S. Army command on 1 July 1973. The new command, along with the U.S. Army Forces Command (FORSCOM), was created from the Continental Army Command (CONARC) located at Fort Monroe, VA. That action was the major innovation in the Army's post-Vietnam reorganization, in the face of realization that CONARC's obligations and span of control were too broad for efficient focus. The new organization functionally realigned the major Army commands in the continental United States. CONARC, and Headquarters, U.S. Army Combat Developments Command (CDC), situated at Fort Belvoir, VA, were discontinued, with TRADOC and FORSCOM at Fort Belvoir assuming the realigned missions. TRADOC assumed the combat developments mission from CDC, took over the individual training mission formerly the responsibility of CONARC, and assumed command from CONARC of the major Army installations in the

---

[2] TRADOC fact sheet available at: http://www.tradoc.army.mil/about.htm

[3] TRADOC commander on ARFORGEN, and the US Army available at: http://www.tradoc.army.mil/about.htm

United States housing Army training center and Army branch schools. FORSCOM assumed CONARC's operational responsibility for the command and readiness of all divisions and corps in the continental U.S. and for the installations where they were based.

Joined under TRADOC, the major Army missions of individual training and combat developments each had its own lineage. The individual training responsibility had belonged, during World War II, to Headquarters Army Ground Forces (AGF). In 1946 numbered Army areas were established in the U.S. under AGF command. At that time, the AGF moved from Washington, D.C. to Fort Monroe, VA. In March 1948, the AGR was replaced at Fort Monroe with the new Office, Chief of Army Field Forces (OCAFF). OCAFF, however, did not command the training establishment. That function was exercised by Headquarters, Department of the Army through the numbered Armies to the corps, division, and Army Training Centers. In February 1955, HQ Continental Army Command (CONARC) replaced OCAFF, assuming its missions as well as the training missions from DA. In January, HQ CONARC was redesignated U.S. Continental Army Command. Combat developments emerged as a formal Army mission in the early 1950s, and OCAFF assumed that role in 1952. In 1955, CONARC assumed the mission. In 1962, HQ U.S. Army Combat Development Command (CDC) was established to bring the combat developments function under one major Army command.[4]

TRADOC Priorities

1. Leader Development
2. Initial Military Training
3. Concepts and Capabilities Integration
4. Human Capital Enterprise
5. Army Training and Learning Concept
6. Doctrine

[4] TRADOC history available at: http://www.tradoc.army.mil/about.htm

Basic Medical Terminology

Subcourse MD0010

This page intentionally left blank.

U. S. ARMY MEDICAL DEPARTMENT CENTER AND SCHOOL
FORT SAM HOUSTON, TEXAS 78234

BASIC MEDICAL TERMINOLOGY

SUBCOURSE MD0010

EDITION 100

DEVELOPMENT

This subcourse is approved for resident and correspondence course instruction. It reflects the current thought of the Academy of Health Sciences and conforms to printed Department of the Army doctrine as closely as currently possible. Development and progress render such doctrine continuously subject to change.

For questions on the content of this subcourse, phone DSN 471-7338 (commercial 210-221-7338), e-mail don.atkerson@amedd.army.mil, or write to:

ACADEMY OF HEALTH SCIENCES
MULTIMEDIA DEVELOPMENT BRANCH
ATTN MCCS HLD
2250 STANLEY ROAD STE 326
FORT SAM HOUSTON TX 78234-6130

ADMINISTRATION

Students who desire credit hours for this correspondence subcourse must meet eligibility requirements and must enroll through the Nonresident Instruction Branch of the U.S. Army Medical Department Center and School (AMEDDC&S).

Initial application for enrollment may be made on DA Form 145 or on ATRRS. If DA Form 145 is used, the approving official must complete the reverse side of the form and forward the form to:

NONRESIDENT INSTRUCTION BRANCH
AMEDDC&S
ATTN: MCCS-HSN
2105 11TH STREET SUITE 4191
FORT SAM HOUSTON TX 78234-6199

or fax the form to 210-221-4012 or DSN 471-4012. A student can self-enroll on ATRRS by going to website http://atrrs.army.mil and submitting the application under the SELF DEVELOPMENT selection.

In general, eligible personnel include enlisted personnel of all components of the U.S. Army who hold an AMEDD MOS (42E, 71G, 76J, and 91-series) or MOS 18D. Officer personnel, members of other branches of the Armed Forces, and civilian employees will be considered for eligibility when the application is authenticated by an approving official and when the requested instruction is job related.

For comments or questions regarding enrollment, student records, or shipments, contact the Nonresident Instruction Branch at DSN 471-5877, commercial (210) 221-5877, toll-free 1-800-344-2380; fax: 210-221-4012 or DSN 471-4012, e-mail accp@amedd.army.mil, or write to the NRIB address given above.

CLARIFICATION OF TRAINING LITERATURE TERMINOLOGY

When used in this publication, words such as "he," "him," "his," and "men" are intended to include both the masculine and feminine genders, unless specifically stated otherwise or when obvious in context.

TABLE OF CONTENTS

CORRESPONDENCE COURSE OF
U.S. ARMY MEDICAL DEPARTMENT CENTER AND SCHOOL

SUBCOURSE MD0010

BASIC MEDICAL TERMINOLOGY

INTRODUCTION

Medical terminology is the professional language of those who are directly or indirectly engaged in the art of healing. You will need to know medical terms in order to read a medical record, to complete forms, to decipher a physician's handwriting, and to communicate with others in the hospital in a professional manner.

At first, the medical terms may seem strange and bewildering to you and appear to be extremely difficult to learn. Fortunately, there is a logical method found in medical terminology. Many of the words used in medicine are made up of parts which are also used in other words. Once you know the meanings of the basic parts of the words, you can put them together to understand the meanings of many medical terms. These basic parts of medical terms are called stems, prefixes, and suffixes. During this course, you will learn to identify and define a stem, a prefix, and a suffix. You will also learn how they are used in combination to describe a medical term.

Subcourse Components:

This subcourse consists of 4 lessons and an examination. The lessons are:

Lesson 1, Introduction to Programmed Learning.

Lesson 2, Stems Pertaining to Medical Terminology.

Lesson 3, Prefixes Pertaining to Medical Terminology.

Lesson 4, Suffixes Pertaining to Medical Terminology.

Examination.

Credit Awarded:

Upon successful completion of this subcourse, you will be awarded 5 credit hours.

Lesson Materials Furnished:

Lesson materials provided include this booklet, an examination answer sheet, and an envelope. Answer sheets are not provided for individual lessons in this subcourse because you are to grade your own lessons. Exercises and solutions for all lessons are contained in this booklet. You must furnish a #2 pencil.

Procedures for Subcourse Completion:

You are encouraged to complete the subcourse lesson by lesson. When you have completed all of the lessons to your satisfaction, fill out the examination answer sheet and mail it to the Army Medical Department Center and School along with the Student Comment Sheet in the envelope provided. Be sure that your social security number is on all correspondence sent to the Army Medical Department Center and School. You will be notified by return mail of the examination results. Your grade on the exam will be your rating for the subcourse.

Purpose:

This programmed instruction subcourse has been prepared for use by students in the medical field. It is designed to help you obtain a knowledge of basic medical terminology. It is NOT intended to be complete or comprehensive. There are numerous textbooks on medical terminology for those students desiring a more complete study of the subject. You are encouraged to continue your study of medical terminology after completing this basic orientation to medical terminology.

This booklet may be written in and retained by the student for future reference. The glossary, pronunciation guide, and list of abbreviations will be a useful reference document.

The final goal or terminal learning objective of this subcourse is that you be able to convert a medical term into lay terminology. This means that when you are given the definition of a medical term, you will be able to identify the proper medical term or, when you are you given the medical term, you will be able to identify the proper definition.

Using the Dictionary:

As you work in the medical field, you will hear and see unfamiliar medical terms. Many times you will have access to a medical dictionary. You need to know how to use a dictionary properly. Most dictionaries have the basic characteristics described below:

a. **Guide Words**. The two large words printed at the top of each page are called "guide words." These words identify the first and last words entered alphabetically on that page, and their use will speed up your process of locating a word. The introduction to the dictionary will tell you how words are alphabetized in that particular dictionary.

b. **Entry**. All the information about a word in the dictionary is called an entry. An entry contains a variety of information and may include all or part of the following information:

(1) Entry word. The entry word is printed in dark type and is sometimes divided into syllables.

(2) Pronunciation. The pronunciation is given in parentheses following the entry word. Different dictionaries use different pronunciation and accent symbols. The introduction portion of each dictionary will provide a key to the symbols.

(3) Plural forms. Frequently, the plural of a medical word is irregularly formed or has alternate plurals. Many medical dictionaries will list these plurals.

(4) Etymology. Etymology is the tracing of a word back to its origins. Information on the origin of the word generally appears in square brackets. Most medical words originated in Greek or Latin or a combination thereof.

(5) Definition. Following the origin, you will find the definition or definitions of the term.

(6) Synonyms. SYN after the definition indicates synonyms. These are words which have a similar meaning to the entry word.

(7) Derived words. Following the SYN, often there is a group of additional words printed in bold type. These words are closely related or derived from the entry words.

(8) Cross reference. For additional information on the term or entry: "See" or "See also," followed by an italicized word, is used.

Introductory Section to a Medical Dictionary:

All dictionaries contain an introductory section which provides information on "how to use" the dictionary. The arrangement of this introduction varies but most medical dictionaries will address the following:

Organization or Arrangement of Entries. This unit addresses how main entries are made, the sequence of entries, and the use of punctuation and capitalization in entries and their sequence.

Pronunciation. This unit provides assistance in pronouncing the word: the diacritical markings (stress marks, long and short vowels, etc.) along with examples of common words to illustrate sounds.

Etymology. A section on the abbreviations used to identify the language of origin along with an explanation of the composition of medical vocabulary is generally included in the introduction. Since more than 75% of medical terms are derived from Latin and Greek, a discussion of the transcription to English of Greek and Latin terms is usually presented. Most sections on etymology include comments on prefixes, suffixes, combining forms, and compounds used in medical terminology. Often the Greek and Latin alphabets are included in the etymology section of the introduction.

Plurals. A presentation on plural forms is included because many plurals are irregularly formed and because many words have alternate plurals. This portion of the introduction will indicate how plurals are presented and listed in the dictionary.

Sample Dictionary Entry:

Appendix (ah-pen'diks), pl. appendixes, appen'dices [L. from appendere to hang upon] a general term used in anatomical nomenclature to designate a supplementary, accessory, or dependent part attached to a main structure; see also appendage. Frequently used alone to refer to the appendix vermiforms.

Appendicopathy (ah-pen"di-kop'ah-the) [appendix + Gr pathos disease] any diseased condition of the vermiform appendix.

Entry word. appendix
appendicopathy

Pronunciation with diacritical markings: ah-pen'diks
ah-pen"di-kop'ah-the

Plural forms: appendixes, appendices

Etymology: [L. from appendere to hang upon] means from the Latin term, appendere, which meant to hang upon.

[appendix + Gr pathos disease] means the stem appendix plus the Greek word pathos which means disease.

Definition: A general term used in anatomical nomenclature to designate a supplementary, accessory, or dependent part attached to a main structure.

Any disease condition of the vermiform appendix.

Synonyms: none

Cross-reference: Appendage.

Refining Your Vocabulary:

This course provides an introduction to the most common medical terms you will encounter. However, just knowing the meaning of the medical terms used in this course is not enough. Developing your medical vocabulary requires refining. As you add words to your medical vocabulary, you must constantly work to use the words correctly. You can refine and sharpen your medical vocabulary through the correct use of a medical dictionary.

Pretest:

This course on medical terminology has one introductory lesson and three lessons related to terminology. Before each lesson, there is a pretest which will enable you to determine your knowledge of medical terminology. You should complete each pretest before working the lesson. If you correctly answer 90% of the pretest questions, you need not work the lesson unless you wish to reinforce your knowledge of medical terminology. The first pretest will test your knowledge of medical stems; the second pretest will test your knowledge of medical prefixes; and the third pretest will test your knowledge of medical suffixes.

Student Comment Sheet:

Be sure to provide us with your suggestions and criticisms by filling out the Student Comment Sheet (found at the back of this booklet), and returning it to us with your examination answer sheet. Please review this comment sheet before studying this subcourse. In this way, you will help us to improve the quality of this subcourse.

LESSON ASSIGNMENT

LESSON 1	Introduction to Programmed Learning.
TEXT ASSIGNMENT	Lesson 1, frame numbers 1-14.
LESSON OBJECTIVE	After completing this lesson, you should be able to: Given a series of frames defining prefix, stem, and suffix, select the correct definition.

LESSON 1

Section I. HOW TO USE PROGRAMMED INSTRUCTION

Directions: Each frame consists of a question and an answer. The answer appears on the right hand side of the page just before the next frame. Make a cover card from a piece of cardboard. Place the cover card over the answer to the frame you are reading. Read the information in the frame and answer the question. Check your answer by moving your cover card down to expose the correct answer.

The programmed instruction format begins on the next page.

GOOD LUCK!

****

1 The material in programmed instruction is arranged in a series of small steps called frames. Each frame presents new information to you or reviews material you may already be familiar with. Therefore, all of the following material is arranged in steps called _________.

frames

****

2 By checking your answer after you have answered a question, you will get immediate feedback as to whether or not you are correct. This immediate feedback will help you learn what is _______________.
(correct, incorrect)

correct

****

3 If your answer is incorrect, you should re-read the frame to find out why you missed the question. Fortunately, all of the information you need to correctly answer the question is contained within that __________.

frame

****

4 Programmed instruction also allows you to learn at your own speed. If the material is difficult for you, you can go slowly. If the material is easy, you can go more ______________.
(slowly, quickly)

quickly

****

****

5 Programmed instruction is designed to proceed logically from one frame to the next frame. When working with programmed instruction, you should not attempt to skip ahead because each frame is developed from preceding frames. That is why this type of material is called _________________________.

programmed instruction

****

Section II. INTRODUCTION TO STEMS, PREFIXES AND SUFFIXES

****

6 All medical terms can be broken down into word parts. The three word parts that you will be concerned with are the prefix, the stem (root), and the suffix. Usually, only two of these parts are present in a medical term. The word parts, then, of a medical term may include the _________, the stem, and the suffix.

prefix

****

7 The stem is the part of the word which gives the basic meaning to the term. The part of the word, "basketball," which gives the basic meaning to the word is "ball." Therefore, "ball" is considered to be the ______.

stem

****

****

8 The part of the word which comes *before* the stem and modifies or augments the meaning of the stem is called the prefix. In the word "basketball," "ball" is the stem and "basket" is the _________________.

prefix

****

9 The part of the word which gives the basic meaning to the word is called the ___________.

stem

****

10 The prefix is the part of the word which comes _________ the stem.
(before, after)

before

****

11 The part of the word which comes *after* the stem and modifies or augments the meaning of the root word is called the suffix. In the term "specialist," "special" is the stem and "ist" is the __________.

suffix

****

12 In summary, words used in medicine are comprised of one or more parts called prefix, stem, and suffix. The part of the word which gives basic meaning to the word is the ______.

stem

****

****

13 The part of the word which comes *before* the stem and modifies or augments the meaning of the stem is called the __________.

prefix

****

14 The part of the word which comes *after* the stem and modifies or augments the meaning of the stem is called the _________.

suffix

****

Now that you're off to a good start, let's look at some medical word parts. BEFORE you look at specific medical word parts, however, you should take the Pretest for lesson 2 on stems which follows this introductory material. Read the Pretest instructions carefully.

Section III. HOW TO COMPLETE EACH PRETEST

1. Before you begin work on your study of medical terminology in lessons 2, 3, and 4, you should complete the pretest for each lesson. The score you make on the pretest will enable you to determine how much you already know about the medical terminology presented in the lesson. The answers to each pretest are found at the end of each lesson. If you score 90% or better on the pretest, it is not necessary for you to work the problems presented in the lesson.

2. If you successfully pass the pretest, you should go to the next pretest. If you successfully pass all the pretests, you should go directly to the final examination.

LESSON ASSIGNMENT

LESSON 2 Stems Pertaining to Medical Terminology.

LESSON ASSIGNMENT Lesson 2, frame numbers 15-131.

LESSON OBJECTIVES After completing this lesson, you should be able to :

2-1. Given a list of 15 of the 100 Latin and Greek medical stems covered in lesson 2 and a list of English meanings for these stems, write the English meaning of the medical stem in the space provided without error.

2-2. Given 10 multiple choice questions on medical stems, select the appropriate English meaning without error.

LESSON 2

PRETEST #1

Before you turn to frame 15 and begin work on your study of medical terminology, complete the pretest on the following pages. The pretest contains 70 questions relating to medical terminology stems. The correct answers to the pretest are found at the end of this lesson. If you correctly answer 90% or more of the questions, you pass the pretest. A score of 90% on this pretest is 63 correct answers.

Write your answers in the space provided in each question.

1. Ophthalmalgia means pain in the __________.

2. Otorrhea is a discharge from the __________.

3. Prenatal means before __________ and post febrile means after __________.

4. A salpingostomy is a surgical opening into a __________.

5. Oophoropexy means fixation of an __________.

6. An enterolith is a __________ in the intestines.

7. Hematuria means the presence of blood in the __________.

8. Orchidectomy means excision of a __________.

9. Cystorrhagia means hemorrhage of the __________.

10. Urethrorrhaphy means suturing the __________.

11. A cholelith is a __________ stone.

12. A hysterosalpingo-oophorectomy means the excision of the __________, __________, and __________.

13. Ureterocele means __________ of the ureter.

14. Esthesia means __________ or __________.

15. Pathophobia means an abnormal __________ of disease.

16. Megalomania is a mental __________.

17. Osteopathy means disease of the __________.

18. Cerebrotomy is an incision into the __________.

19. Neuralgia means pain along the course of a __________.

20. Glycolysis is the breakdown or destruction of __________.

21. Edema means __________.

22. Acroparalysis refers to paralysis of the __________.

23. Tachyphagia is a word for fast or rapid __________.

24. Splenopathy means a disease of the __________.

25. Lymphostasis means control the flow of __________.

26. An encephaloma is a __________.

27. Lipolysis means destruction or breakdown of __________.

28. A pyocele is a hernia containing __________.

29. Dacryorrhea means excessive flow of __________.

30. Cytology is the study of __________.

31. Thrombus is the medical way to say __________.

32. Arterioplasty is surgical repair of an __________.

33. Phlebosclerosis is the hardening of the __________.

34. Vasotripsy means the crushing of a __________.

35. An angiospasm is a spasm of a __________.

36. Hepatomegaly means enlargement of the __________.

37. A proctoscopy is an examination of the __________.

38. Colocentesis means puncture of the __________.

39. Jejunoileitis is inflammation of the __________ and the __________.

40. Psychosis means any serious __________ condition.

41. Enteroptosis means prolapse of the small __________.

42. Gastrectasia is the dilation or stretching of the __________.

43. Gingivalgia means pain in the __________.

44. The lacrimal gland secretes __________.

45. Cheilosis is a disorder of the __________.

46. A duodenotomy is an incision into the __________.

47. Stomatoplasty means surgical repair of the __________.

48. Apnea means temporary cessation of __________.

49. Treatment with compressed __________ is called pneumotherapy.

50. A laparorrhaphy is the suturing of the __________.

51. Glossoplegia is a paralysis of the __________.

52. Bronchorrhagia means __________hemorrhage.

53. Nasal means pertaining to the __________.

54. Rhinoplasty means surgical repair of the __________.

55. Laryngitis is inflammation of the __________.

56. Onychosis means a condition of the __________.

57. Costal means pertaining to the __________.

58. Abdominocentesis is a surgical puncture of the __________.

59. Tendinitis is inflammation of the __________.

60. Myocarditis is inflammation of the heart __________.

61. Myelocele means herniation of the __________ __________.

62. Chondromalacia is the softening of __________.

63. Arthritis is a word which means inflammation of a__________.

64. A tympanectomy is an excision of the __________.

65. Keratectasia means dilatation of the __________.

66. A pharyngotomy is an incision into the __________.

67. Blepharoptosis means prolapse of the __________.

68. Hemostasis means the act of controlling the flow of __________.

69. A necroparasite is one that lives on __________ organic matter.

70. Pneumomycosis is a condition of lung __________.

Check your answers on page 2-77

Section II. BASIC COMPONENTS

NOTE: Please refer to the pronunciation guide on page B-1 to assist you in pronouncing the terms you will encounter in this lesson.

We will first discuss the main body or basic component of a medical term called the stem or root word. The stem of a medical word usually indicates the organ or part which is modified by a prefix or suffix, or both.

****

15. The main body or basic component of a word is called the ______ or _______ word.

stem root

****

16. All words have a stem. Even everyday words have stems. For example, in the words "singer," "writer," and "speaker," "sing," "write," and "speak" are the stems. In medical terms such as hepatomone, gastrotome, and arthrotome, the <u>hepat</u> (meaning liver), <u>gastr</u> (meaning stomach), and <u>arthr</u> (meaning joint) are the ___________.

stems

****

17. Certain combinations of stems are hard to pronounce. This is often true when a stem ends in a consonant and the word part that is added to it also begins with a consonant. This awkwardness of pronunciation makes it necessary to insert a vowel called a combining vowel.

****

18. Certain combinations of stems or root words are difficult to pronounce, making it necessary to insert a vowel called a ________________.

combining vowel

****

19. Usually the combining vowel is an "o," but occasionally it may be "a," "e," "i," "u," or "y."

****

20. The combining vowel is usually an ______________.

o

****

21. We find combining vowels in ordinary words. Instead of joining the two stems "therm" and "meter" directly, we insert the combining vowel "o" and say "therm - 'o' meter."

****

22. Here are some more examples:

a. Speed - meter becomes speed-ometer.
b. Megal - mania becomes mega-lomania.
c. Strat - phere becomes strato-sphere.
d. Therm - meter becomes ther-mometer.

****

23. Instead of joining two stems or root words directly, we insert the combining vowel which is usually an __________.

o

****

24. A stem plus the combining vowel is known as the combining form.

In the word speedometer, for example, "speed" is the stem and "speed -o" is the combining form.

****

25. In the word thermometer, "therm" is the stem and "therm - o" is the

_________________.

combining form

****

26. In the word megalomania, "megal" is the stem and "megal - o" is

_________________.

combining form

****

27. In the word stratosphere, "strat" is the stem and "strat- o" is the

________________.

combining form

****

28. As a review, complete each of the following statements:

a. The basic core of any word is the ________.

stem (frame 15)

****

b. Combinations of stems are often difficult to pronounce. When the first stem ends in a consonant and the second word part begins with a consonant, we must insert a vowel called a __________ vowel.

combining (frame 17)

****

c. The combining vowel is usually an _______.

o (frame 19)

****

d. The combination of a stem plus a combining vowel is known as the ______________.

combining form (frame 24)

****

NOTE: Each frame which introduces a new medical term contains the correct pronunciation with diacritical markings. The pronunciation guide below should be used to help you pronounce the medical term correctly. You should pronounce each medical term aloud so that you can hear how the word sounds. Practicing the correct pronunciation aloud will also help you remember the term and its meaning.

USE THIS GUIDE TO ASSIST YOU IN PRONUNCIATION

IF IT IS AN	AND	THEN IT IS
UNMARKED VOWEL	IT ENDS A SYLLABLE	LONG "ā" (UNLESS OTHERWISE INDICATED)
	THE SYLLABLE ENDS IN A CONSONANT	SHORT "ă" (UNLESS OTHERWISE INDICATED)

In this course, stems are presented with the combining vowel and in their combining forms (stem + combining vowel = combining form) and referred to simply as the stem.

Although Latin combining forms (stem + combining vowel) should be used only with Latin prefixes and suffixes and Greek combining forms with Greek pre-fixes and suffixes, there are generally many inconsistencies in forming medical terms.

The combining forms presented in this text are legitimate; however, you will not find all the combining forms used in this text in any one medical dictionary. The combining form of the stem, tendo, for example does not appear in some dictionaries and appears in different forms in other medical dictionaries as follows:

Stedman's Medical Dictionary - tendo-. Combining form meaning tendon; see also teno-. Teno-, tenon-, tenonto-. Combining forms meaning tendon. See also tendo-.

Blakinton's Gould Medical Dictionary - ten-, teno-. A combining form meaning tendon.

Dorland's Illustrated Medical Dictionary - teno-, tenonto-. Combining form denoting relationship to a tendon.

Several sources were used as references in compiling the information included in this text including the following:

Dorland's Illustrated Medical Dictionary.
Blakinton's Gould Medical Dictionary.
Stedman's Medical Dictionary.
Taber's Cyclopedic Medical Dictionary.

Section III. STEMS - PERTAINING TO THE MUSCULOSKELETAL SYSTEM

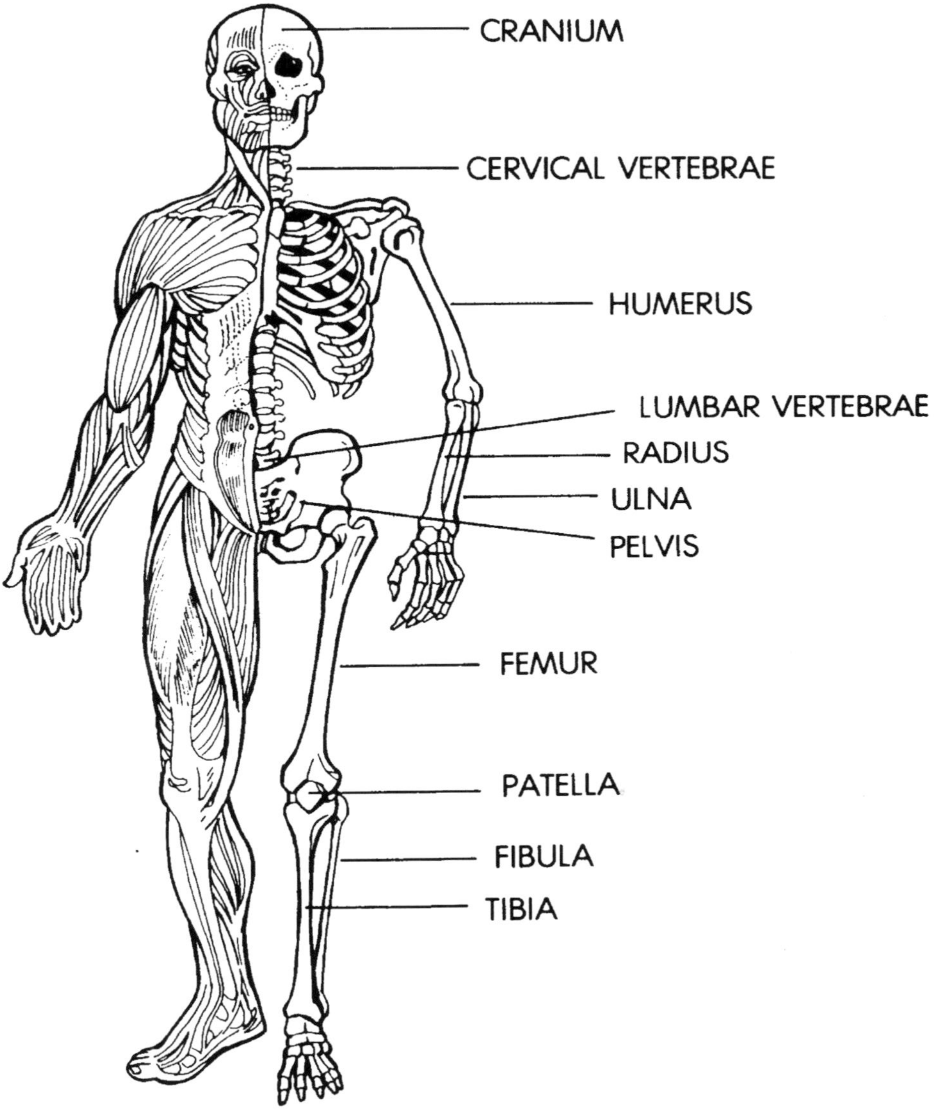

Now let's look at some of the more common stems pertaining to the musculoskeletal system.

****

29. The musculoskeletal system includes the bones, muscles, and joints.

****

30. Osteo is a stem which means bone. A person who has osteo-arthritis, for example, has inflammation of the ______ and joint.

os"te-o-ar-thri'-tis

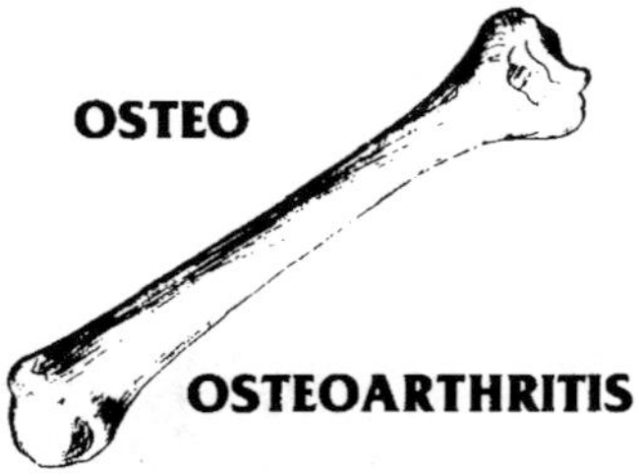

bone

****

31. The stem, arthro, means joint. Arthrodesis means fixation of a _______ by fusion.

ar"thro-de'-sis

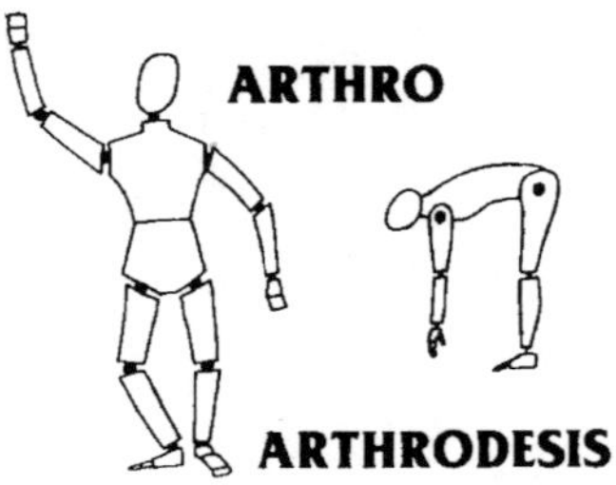

joint

****

32. The stem chondro means cartilage. A person with chondr-itis, for example, has inflammation of the _________.

kon-dri'tis

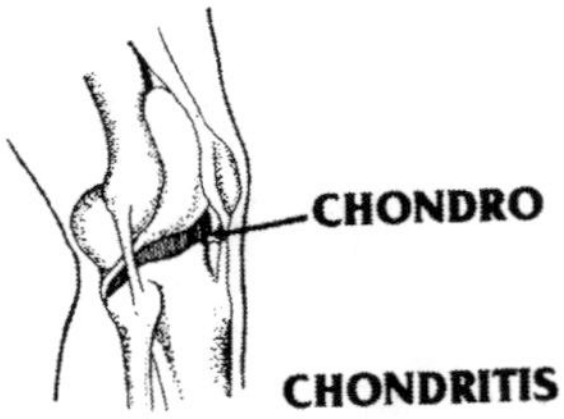

cartilage

****

33. The stem myelo means bone marrow or spine. A person who has myelitis has an inflammation of the _______ ________ or _________.

mi"e-li'tis

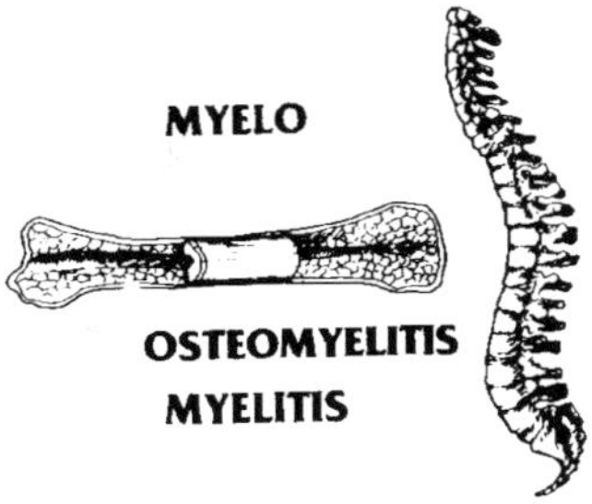

bone marrow/spine

****

34. Myo is a stem which means muscle. A myospasm, for example, is an involuntary contraction of a ___________.

mi'o-spazm

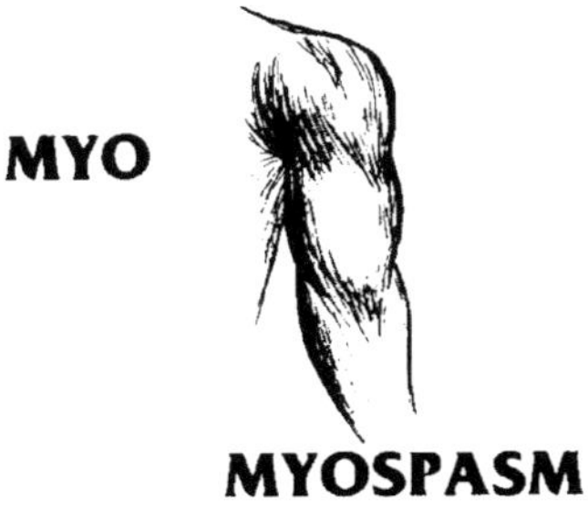

muscle

****

35. Tendo is a stem which means tendon. A person with tend-initis has inflammation of a _________.

ten"di-ni'tis

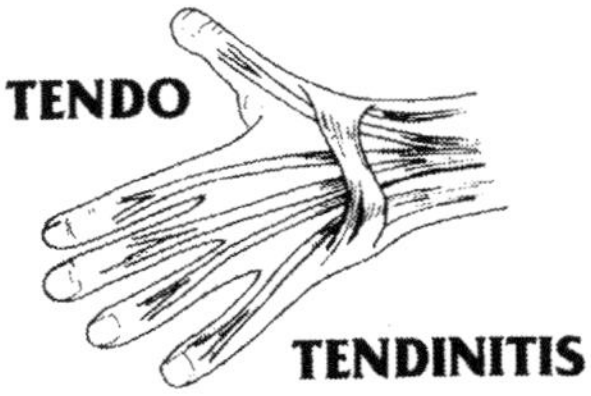

tendon

****

36. Costo is a stem which means rib. The intercostal space, for example, refers to the space between the ___________.

in"ter-kos'tal

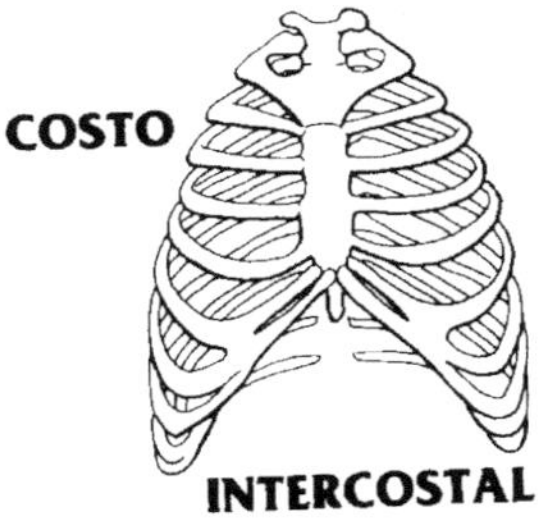

ribs

****

37. As a review, give the meaning of each of the following stems pertaining to the musculoskeletal system.

a. Osteo: _________

bone (frame 30)

****

b. Arthro: _________

joint (frame 31)

****

c. Chondro: _________

cartilage (frame 32)

****

d. Myelo: _________

bone marrow/spine (frame 33)

****

e. Myo: _________

muscle (frame 34)

****

f. Tendo: _________

tendon (frame 35)

****

g. Costo: _________

rib (frame 36)

****

38. To further reinforce what you have learned, fill in the blanks with the appropriate words:

a. A person who has osteoarthritis has inflammation of the ______ and _________.

bone/joint (frames 30 & 31)

****

b. Arthrodesis is fixation of a __________ by fusion.

joint (frame 31)

****

c. A person with chondritis has inflammation of the __________.

cartilage (frame 32)

****

d. A person who has myelitis has inflammation of the _____ _______ or __________.

bone marrow/spine (frame 33)

****

e. A myospasm is an involuntary contraction of a __________.

muscle (frame 34)

****

f. A person with tendinitis has an inflammation of a __________.

tendon (frame 35)

****

g. Intercostal refers to the space between the __________.

ribs (frame 36)

****

If you missed any of the questions in frames 37 and 38, please review the appropriate frame(s) before continuing to frame 39.

Section IV. STEMS - PERTAINING TO THE INTEGUMENTARY SYSTEM

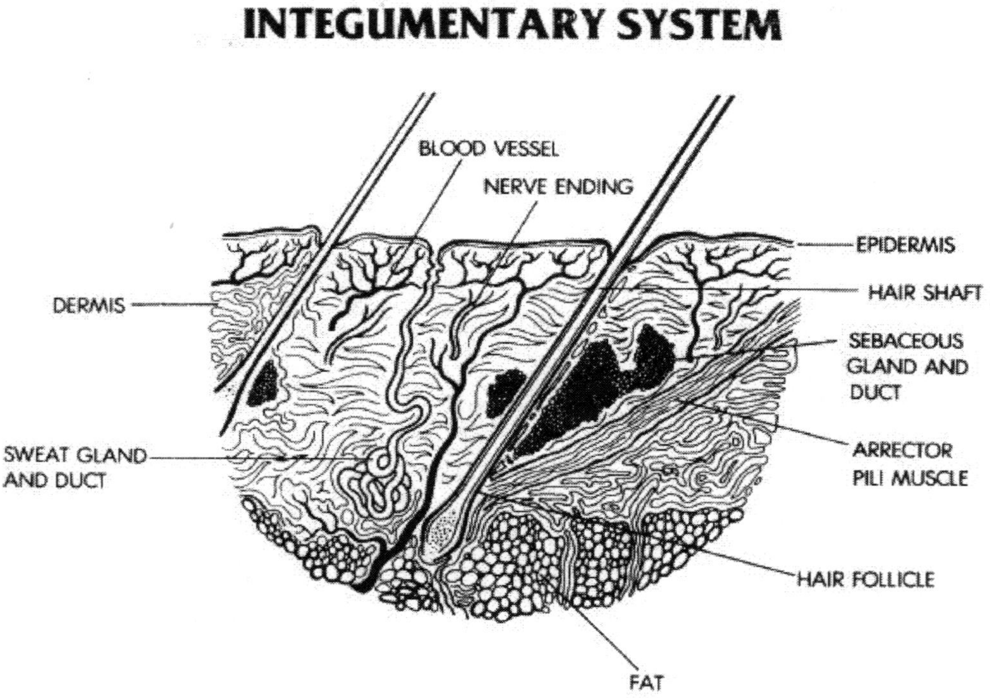

The integumentary system includes the skin and its appendages - the hair and nails.

39. Derma is a stem which means skin. A person with dermatophytosis, for example, has a fungus condition of the __________.

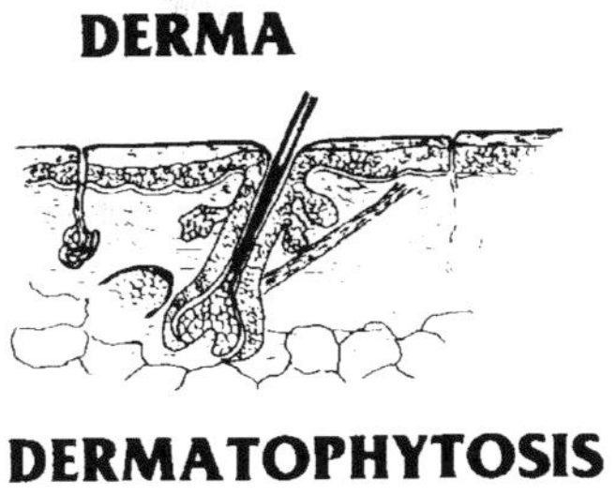

der"mah-to-fi-to'sis

skin

****

40. Onycho is a stem which means nail. Onychectomy means surgical removal of the _________of a finger or toe.

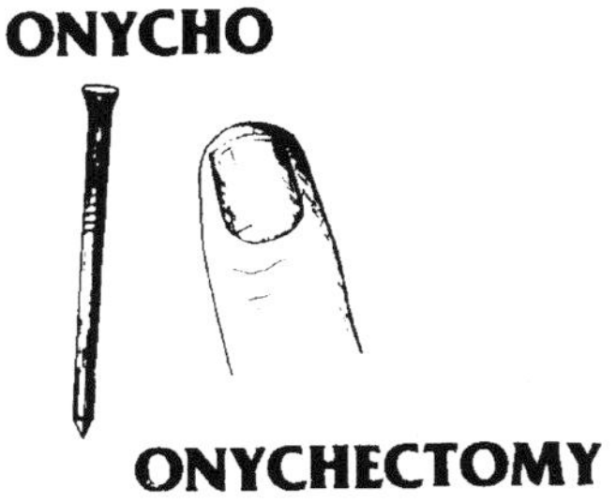

on"i-kek'to-me

nail

****

41. Let's review the stems you've just studied. Give the meaning of each of the following stems pertaining to the integumentary system:

a. Derma: __________

skin (frame 39)

****

b. Onycho: __________

nail (frame 40)

****

42. Let's make sure you know the stems you have just studied. Fill in the blanks with the appropriate terms.

a. A person with dermatophytosis has a fungus condition of the __________.

skin (frame 39)

****

b. Onychectomy is the surgical removal of the __________ of a finger or toe.

nail (frame 40)

****

If you missed any of the questions in frames 41 and 42, please review the appropriate frame(s) before continuing to frame 43.

Section V. STEMS - PERTAINING TO THE RESPIRATORY SYSTEM

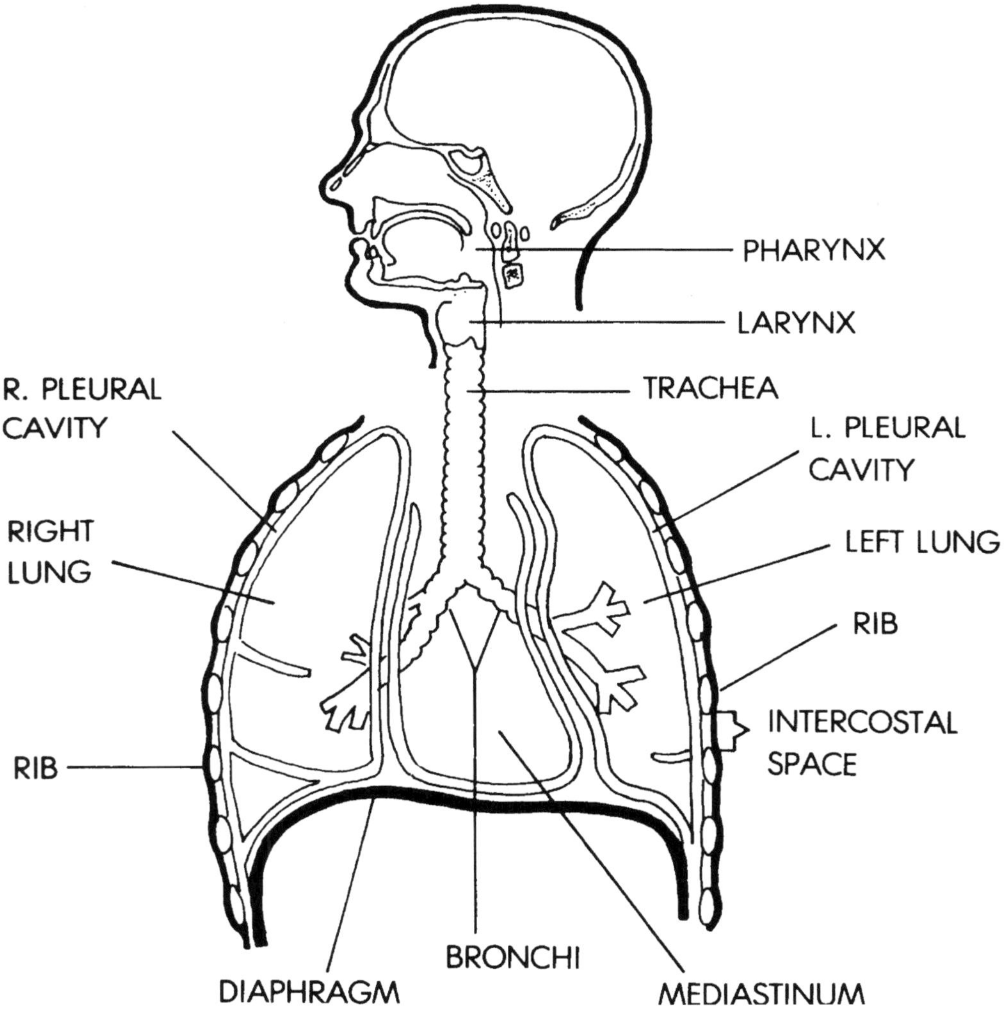

The respiratory system includes the lungs, pleura, bronchi, pharynx, larynx, tonsils, and the nose.

43. Rhino and naso are stems which mean nose. A person who has rhinitis has inflammation of the __________.

ri-ni'tis

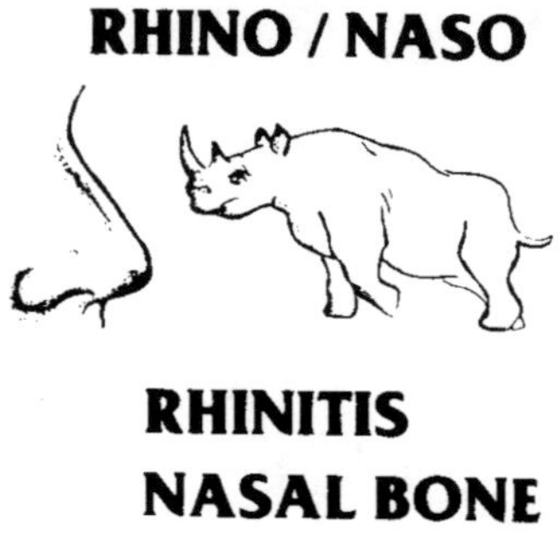

nose

****

44. Laryngo is a stem meaning larynx or voice box. A laryngoscopy is an examination of the interior of the __________.

lar"ing-gos'ko-pe

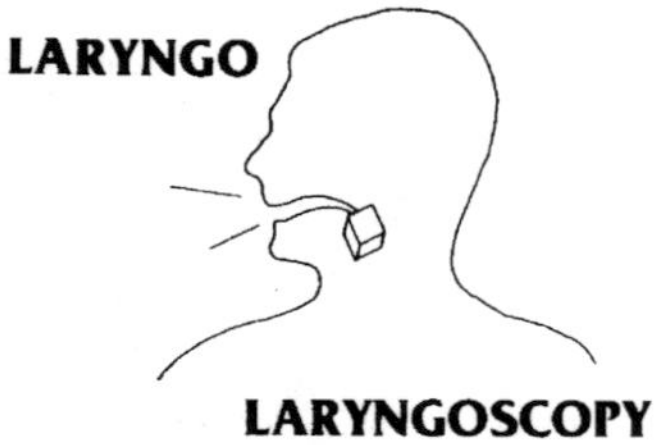

larynx

****

45. Tracheo is a stem which means upper windpipe or trachea. A person with tracheitis has an inflammation of the __________ __________ or __________.

tra"ke-i'tis

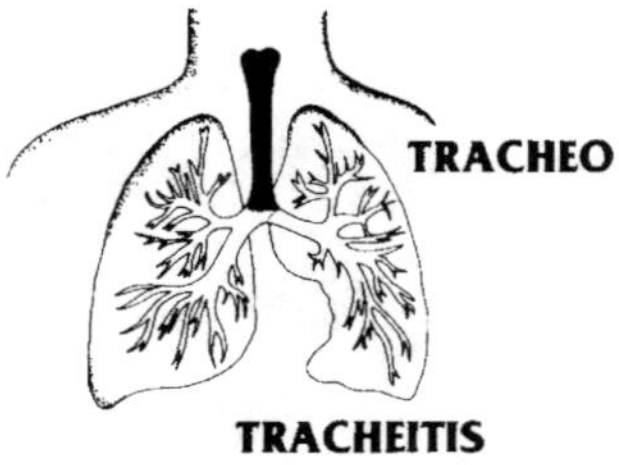

upper windpipe/trachea

****

46. Broncho is a stem which means lower windpipe or bronchus. A person with bronchitis has inflammation of the __________ __________ or __________.

brong-ki'tis

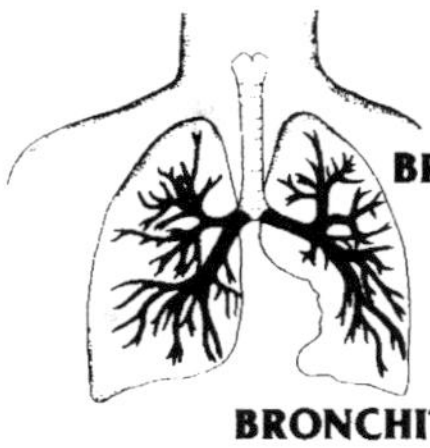

lower windpipe/bronchus

****

47. Pulmo and pneumo are stems which mean lung. Pulmonary, for example, means concerning or involving the __________.

pul'mo-ner"e

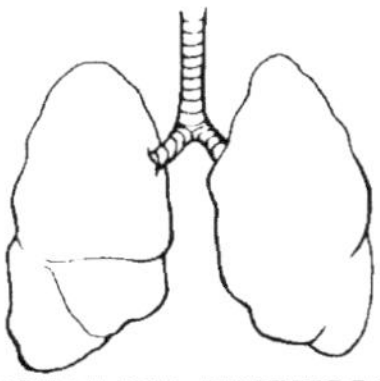

lungs

****

48. A person with pneumonia has an inflammation of the __________.

nu-mo'ne-ah

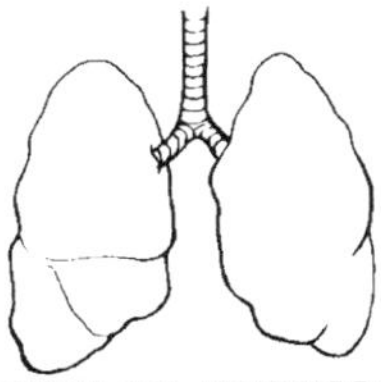

lungs

****

49. Pneumo is a stem which also means air. Pneumonemia is the presence of ________ or gas in the blood vessel.

nu"mo-ne'me-ah

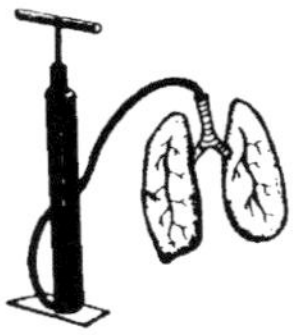

air

****

50. Pneo is a stem which means breath or breathing. Pneodynamics is the mechanism of __________.

ne'o-di nam'ik

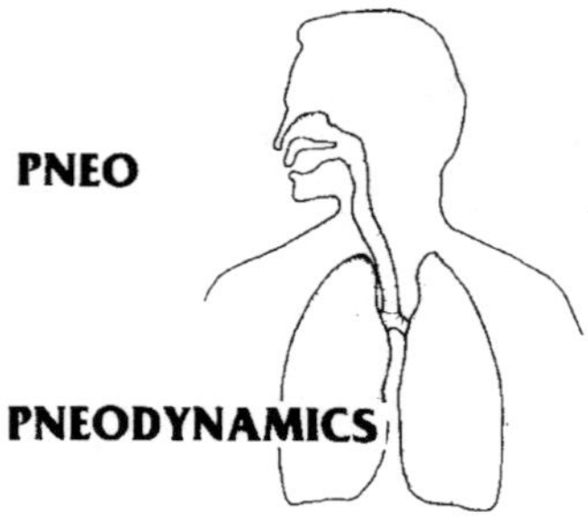

breathing

****

51. Let's review the stems you just studied. Give the meaning of each of the following stems pertaining to the respiratory system.

a. Rhino: __________

nose (frame 43)

****

b. Naso: __________

nose (frame 43)

****

c. Laryngo: __________

larynx (frame 44)

****

d. Tracheo: __________ __________ or __________

upper windpipe/trachea (frame 45)

****

e. Broncho: __________ __________ or __________

lower windpipe/bronchus (frame 46)

****

f. Pulmo: __________

lung (frame 47)

****

g. Pneumo: _______ or _______

air/lungs (frame 47/49)

****

h. Pneo: __________

breathing (frame 50)

****

52. To further reinforce what you have learned, fill in the blanks with the appropriate terms:

a. A person who has rhinitis has an inflammation of the __________.

nose (frame 43)

****

b. A laryngoscope is an instrument used for examination of the __________.

larynx (frame 44)

****

c. Tracheitis is the inflammation of the _______ _______ or _________.

upper windpipe/trachea (frame 45)

****

d. A child who has bronchitis has an inflammation of the _______ _______ or __________.

lower windpipe/bronchus (frame 46)

****

e. The pulmonary artery leads to the __________.

lungs (frame 47)

****

f. A person with pneumonia has an inflammation of the __________.

lungs (frame 48)

****

g. Pneumonemia is the presence of __________ or gas in the blood vessels.

air (frame 49)

****

h. Pneodynamics is the mechanism of __________.

breathing (frame 50)

****

If you missed any of the questions in frames 51 and 52, please review the appropriate frame(s) before continuing to frame 53.

Section VI: STEMS - PERTAINING TO THE DIGESTIVE SYSTEM

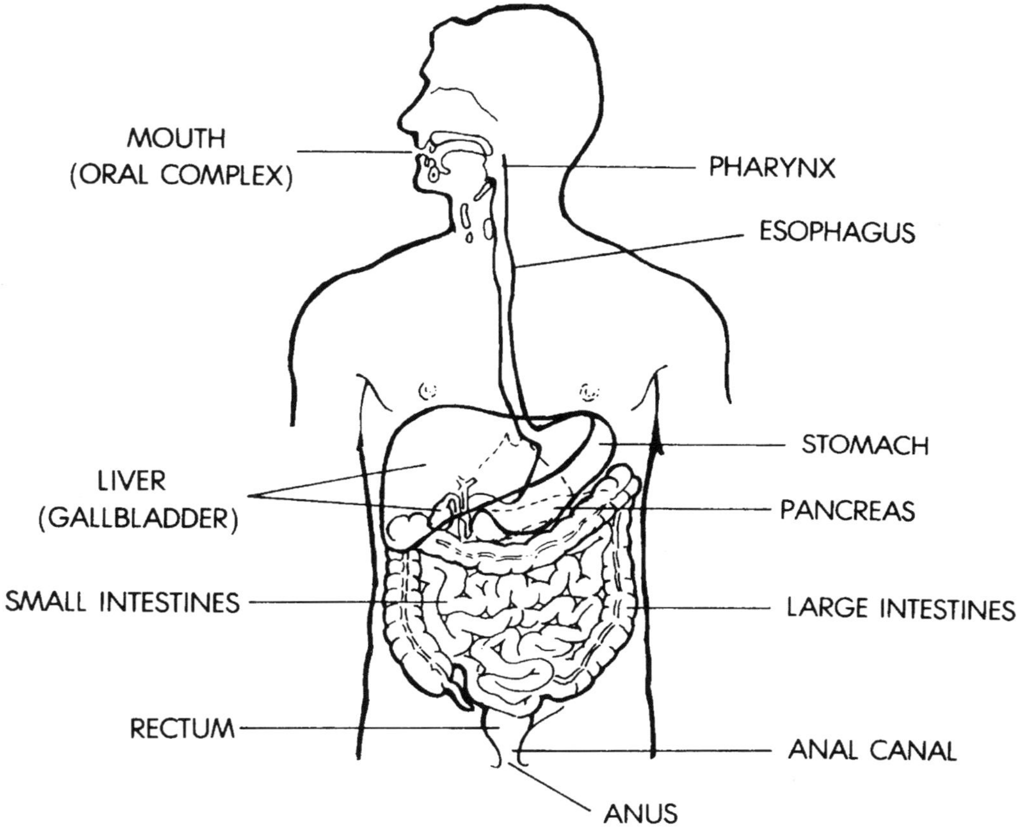

The digestive system or gastrointestinal tract begins with the mouth, where food enters the body and ends with the anus, where solid waste material leaves the body.

****

53. The stem stoma means mouth. A person who has stomatitis, for example, has inflammation of the __________.

sto-mah-ti'tis

STOMA

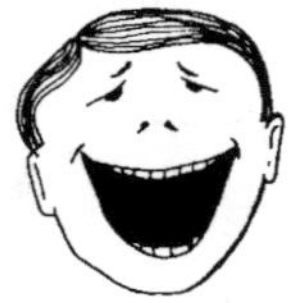

STOMATITIS

mouth

****

54. Lingua and glossa are stems which mean tongue. Glossitis means inflammation of the __________.

glos-si'tis

LINGUA / GLOSSA

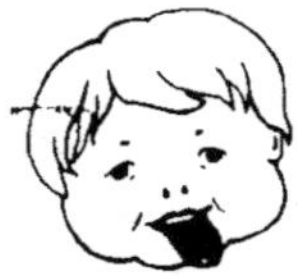

LINGUAL / GLOSSITIS

tongue

****

55. Lingual means pertaining to the __________.

ling'gwal

LINGUA / GLOSSA

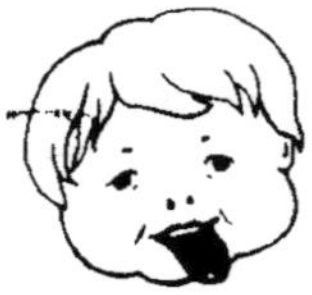

LINGUAL / GLOSSITIS

tongue

****

56. Dento and odonto are stems which mean tooth. A person with dentalgia has a pain in the __________.

den-tal'je-ah

DENTO / ODONTO

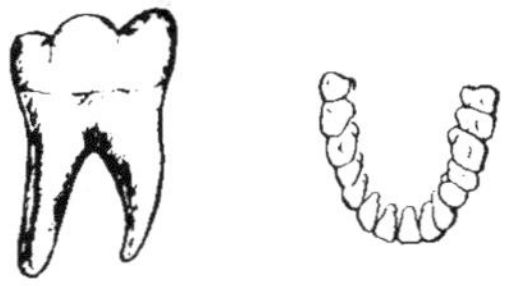

DENTALGIA

ODONTOID

tooth

****

57. Cheilo is a stem which means lip. A cheiloplasty is the surgical repair of a defect of the __________.

ki'lo-plas"te

CHEILO

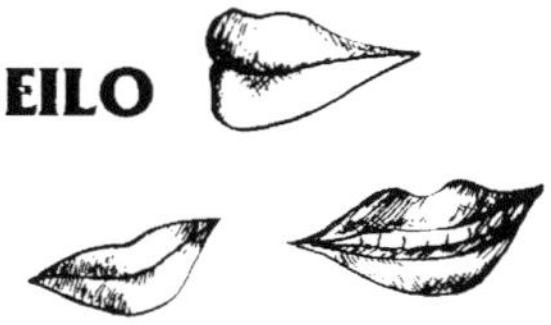

CHEILOPLASTY

lip

****

58. Gingivo is a stem which means gums. A person with gingivitis has an inflammation of the __________.

jin"ji-vi'tis

GINGIVO

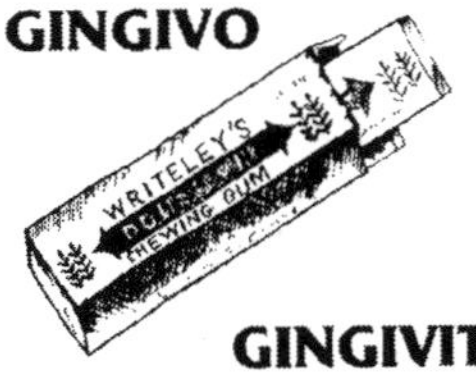

GINGIVITIS

gums

****

59. Gastro is a stem which means stomach. A gastrectomy is the surgical removal of the __________.

gas-trek-to-me

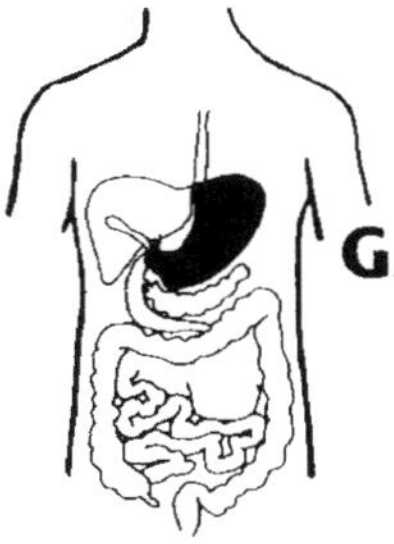

GASTRO

GASTRECTOMY

stomach

****

60. Entero is a stem which means intestine. A person with gastroenteritis has inflammation of the stomach and __________.

gas"tro-en-ter-i'tis

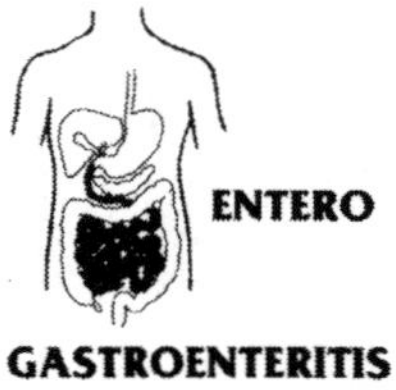

intestine

****

61. Duodeno is a stem which pertains to the duodenum or first part of the small intestine. A duodenal ulcer, for example, is an ulcer which is located in the __________ or ______________________________.

du"o-de'nal

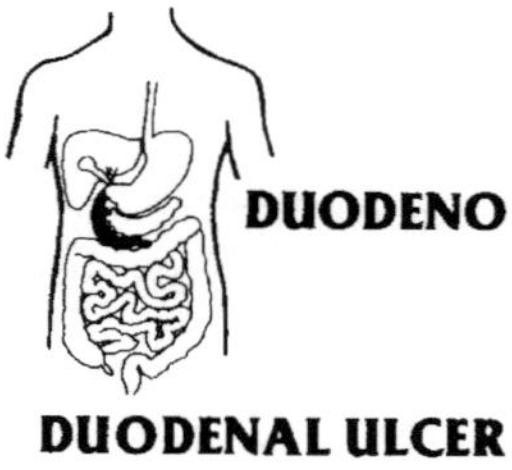

duodenum or first part of the small intestine

****

62. Jejuno is a stem which pertains to the jejunum or second part of the small intestine. A jejunectomy, for example, is an excision of a part of or all of the __________ or __________.

je-joo'num
je"joo-nek'to-me

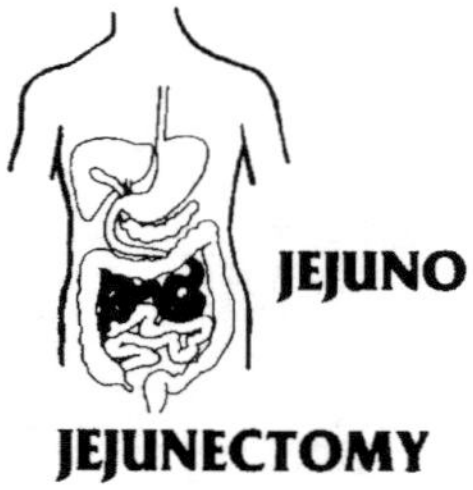

jejunum or second part of the small intestine

****

63. Ileo is a stem which pertains to the ileum or third part of the small intestine. Ileitis means inflammation of the __________ or ____________________.

il'e-um
il"e-i'tis

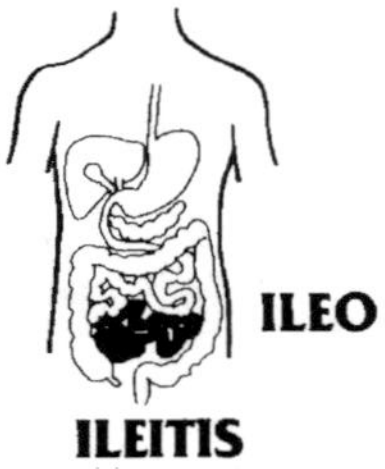

ileum or third part of the small intestine

****

64. Colo is a stem which means colon. When a colostomy is performed, an incision is made into the _________.

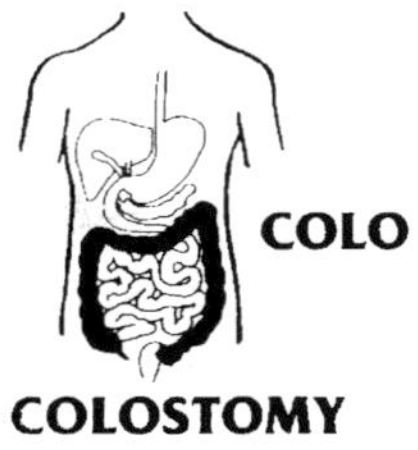

ko'lon
ko-los'to-me

colon

****

65. Procto and ano are stems which mean rectum or anus. Proctitis means inflammation of the ________ or _________.

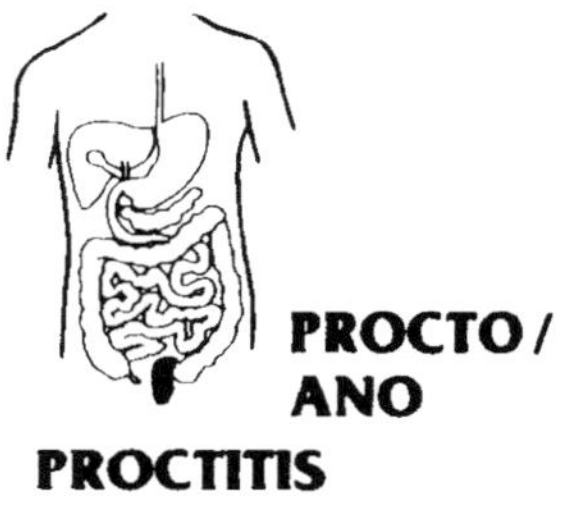

prok-ti'tis

rectum or anus

****

66. As a review, give the meaning of the following stems pertaining to the digestive system.

a. Stoma: __________

mouth (frame 53)

****

b. Lingua/glossa: __________

tongue (frame 54)

****

c. Dento/odonto: __________

tooth (frame 56)

****

d. Cheilo: _________

lip (frame 57)

****

e. Gingivo: __________

gums (frame 58)

****

f. Gastro: __________

stomach (frame 59)

****

g. Entero: __________

intestine (frame 60)

****

h. Duodeno: __________

duodenum/first part of intestine (frame 61)

****

i. Jejuno: __________

jejunum/2d part of intestine (frame 62)

****

j. Ileo: __________

ileum/3d part of intestine (frame 63)

****

k. Colo: __________

colon (frame 64)

****

l. Procto/ano: __________

rectum/anus

****

67. Fill in the blanks with the appropriate terms:

a. A person with stomatitis has an inflammation of the __________.

mouth (frame 53)

****

b. Glossitis is an inflammation of the __________.

tongue (frame 54)

****

c. Lingual means pertaining to the __________.

tongue (frame 54)

****

d. A person with dentalgia has a pain in the __________.

tooth (frame 56)

****

e. A cheiloplasty is the surgical repair of a defect of the __________.

lip (frame 57)

****

f. Someone who has gingivitis has inflammation of the __________.

gums (frame 58)

****

g. A gastrectomy is the surgical removal of the __________.

stomach (frame 59)

****

h. A person with gastroenteritis has inflammation of the __________ and the __________.

stomach and intestine(frames 59 & 60)

****

i. A duodenal ulcer is located in the __________.

duodenum/1st part of the small intestine (frame 61)

****

j. A jejunectomy is an excision of part or all of the ______________.

jejunum/2d part of the small intestine (frame 62)

****

k. Ileitis is an inflammation of the ______________.

ileum/3d part of the small intestine (frame 63)

****

l. A colostomy is an incision into the
___________.

colon (frame 64)

****

m. Proctitis is an inflammation of the
___________ or ___________.

rectum/anus (frame 65)

****

If you missed any of the questions in frames 66 and 67, please review the appropriate frame(s) before continuing to frame 68.

Section VII. STEMS - PERTAINING TO THE ACCESSORY ORGANS OF DIGESTION

****

68. The stem hepato means liver. A person with hepatitis has an inflammation of the __________.

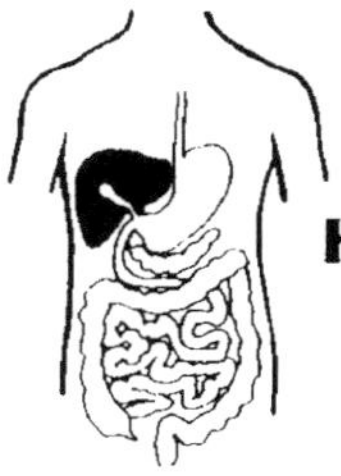

HEPATO

hep"ah-ti'tis

HEPATITIS

liver

****

69. The stem cholecysto means gall-bladder. A person who has had an operation called a cholecystectomy, for example, has had his _____________ removed (or excised).

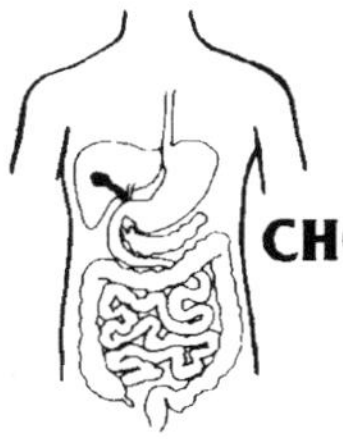

CHOLECYSTO

ko"le-sis-tek'to-me

CHOLECYSTECTOMY

gallbladder

****

70. The stems celio and abdomino mean abdomen. A person who has had a celiectomy has had a complete or partial removal of an organ of the __________.

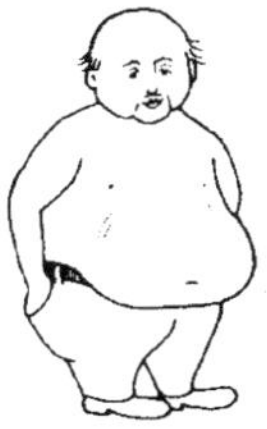

CELIO / ABDOMINO

se"le-ek'to-me

CELIECTOMY
ABDOMINAL

abdomen

****

71. Laparo is a stem meaning abdominal wall. A person who has a laparotomy has had an incision made into the

__________ __________.

lap-ah-rot'o-me

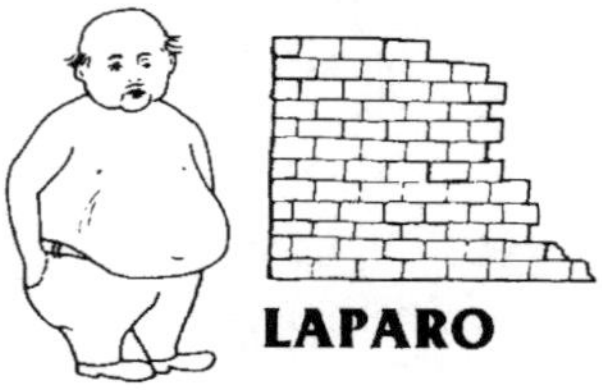

LAPAROTOMY

abdominal wall

****

72. As a review, give the meaning of each of the following terms:

a. Hepato: __________

liver (frame 68)

****

b. Cholecysto: __________

gallbladder (frame 69)

****

c. Celio/abdomino: __________

abdomen (frame 70)

****

d. Laparo: __________

abdominal wall (frame 71)

****

73. To further reinforce what you have learned, fill in the blanks with the appropriate terms:

a. A person who has hepatitis has an inflammation of the __________.

liver (frame 68)

****

b. When a cholecystectomy is performed, the __________ is removed (or excised).

gallbladder (frame 69)

****

c. A person who has a celiectomy has had a complete or partial removal of an organ of the

___________.

abdomen (frame 70)

****

d. During a laparotomy, an incision is made into the ___________.

abdominal wall (frame 71)

****

If you missed any of the questions in frames 72 and 73, please review the appropriate frame(s) before continuing to frame 74.

Section VIII. STEMS - PERTAINING TO THE CARDIOVASCULAR SYSTEM

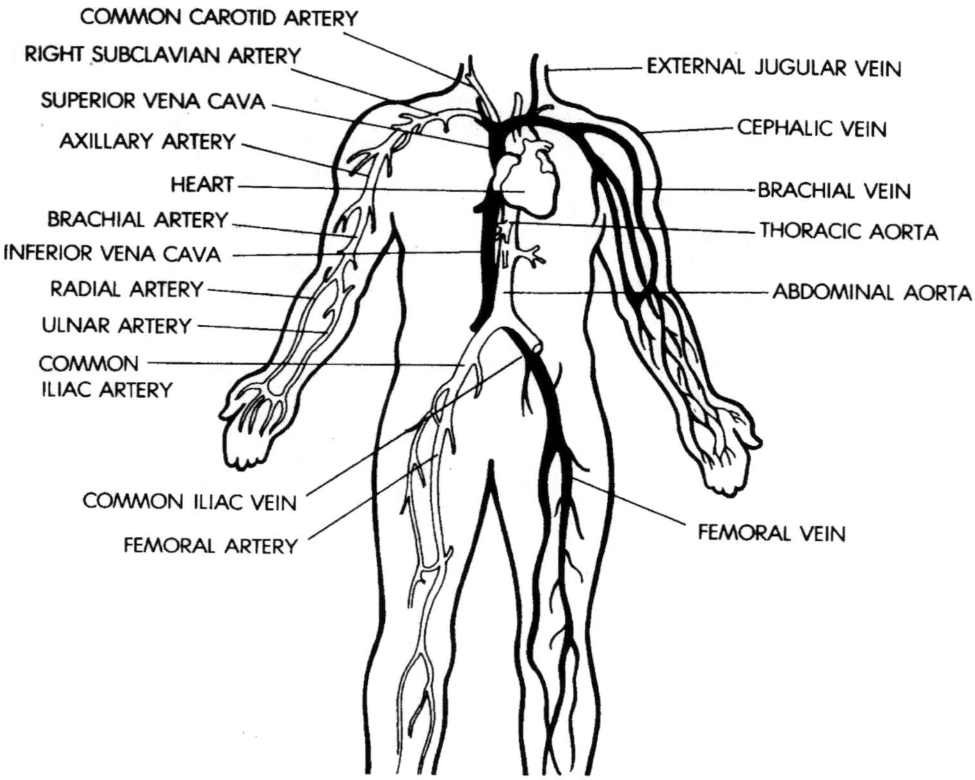

The cardiovascular system includes the heart and blood vessels.

****

74. The stem, <u>cardio</u>, means heart. The <u>cardio</u>vascular system includes the blood vessels and the __________.

kar"de-o-vas'ku-lar

CARDIO

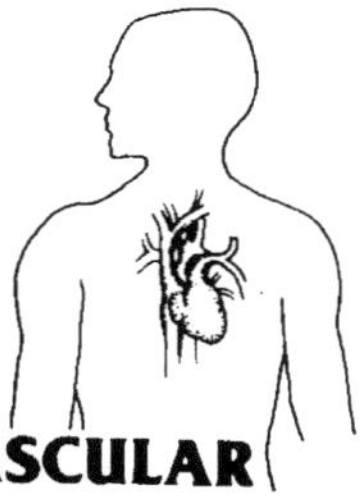

CARDIOVASCULAR

heart

****

75. <u>Angio</u> and <u>vaso</u> are stems which mean vessel. An <u>angio</u>gram is a series of X-ray film of a blood __________.

an'je-o-gram"

ANGIO / VASO

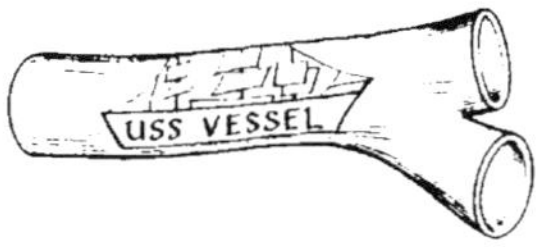

ANGIOGRAM / VASODILATOR

vessel

****

76. <u>Phlebo</u> and <u>veno</u> are stems which mean vein. A <u>phleb</u>ectomy is the surgical removal of a __________.

fle-bek'to-me

PHLEBO / VENO

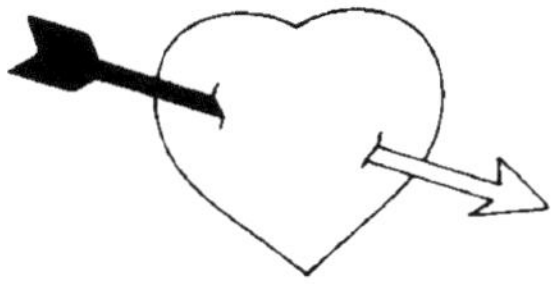

PHLEBECTOMY
VENOGRAM

vein

****

77. Arterio is a stem which means artery. A person who has arteriosclerosis has hardening of the __________.

ar-te"re-o-skle-ro'sis

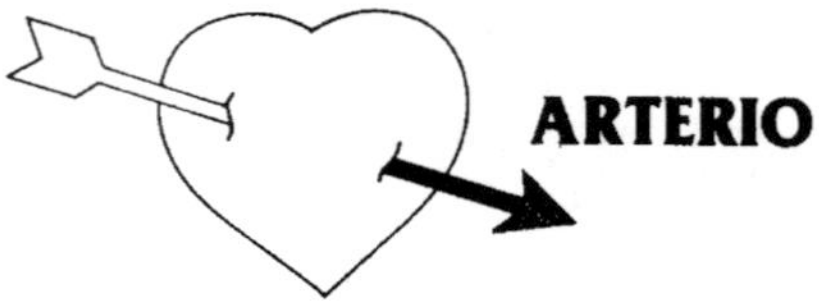

ARTERIOSCLEROSIS

arteries

****

78. Thrombo is a stem which means clot of blood. Thrombophlebitis is an inflammation of a vein with a __________ of __________.

throm"bo-fle-bi'tis

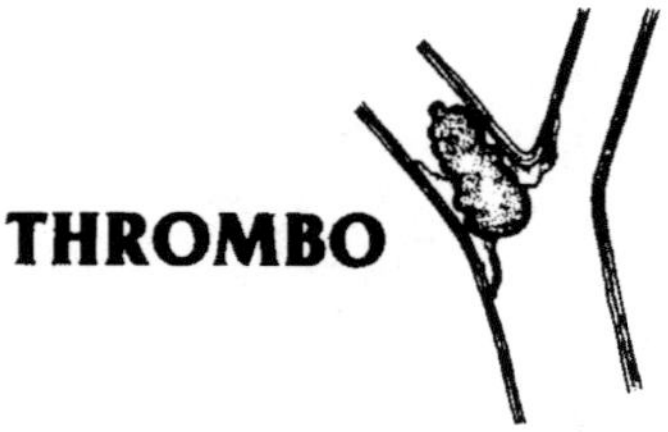

THROMBOPHLEBITIS

clot/blood

****

79. As a review, give the meaning of each of the following terms pertaining to the cardiovascular system.

a. cardio: __________

heart (frame 74)

****

b. angio/vaso: __________

vessel (frame 75)

****

c. phlebo/veno: __________

vein (frame 76)

****

d. arterio: __________

artery (frame 77)

****

e. thrombo: __________

clot of blood (frame 78)

****

80. To further reinforce what you have learned, fill in the blanks with the appropriate terms:

a. The cardiovascular system includes the blood vessels and the __________.

heart (frame 74)

****

b. When a person has an angiospasm or a vasospasm, he has a spasm of a __________.

vessel (frame 75)

****

c. A phlebectomy is the surgical removal of a __________.

vein (frame 76)

****

d. A person who has arteriomalacia has a softening of the __________.

arteries (frame 77)

****

e. A thrombectomy is the excision of a __________.

clot of blood (frame 78)

****

If you missed any of the questions in frames 79 and 80, please review the appropriate frame(s) before continuing to frame 81.

Section IX. STEMS - PERTAINING TO THE HEMATOPOIETIC AND LYMPATHIC SYSTEMS

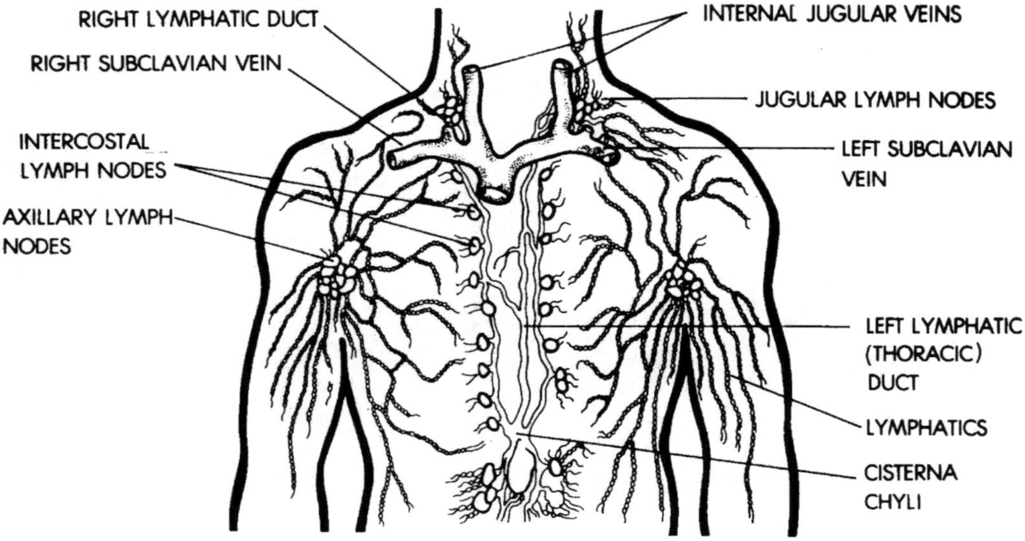

The hematopoietic system includes tissues concerned in the production of blood. The lymphatic system includes the lymphatic vessels and lymphoid tissues.

****

81. Cyto is a stem meaning cell. An erythrocyte is one kind of blood cell. It is a red blood __________.

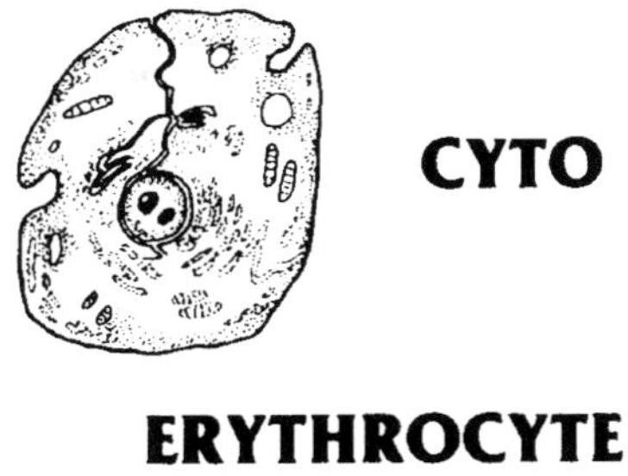

e-rith'ro-sit

cell

****

82. Hema and hemato are stems which mean blood. A hematoma is a tumor filled with __________.

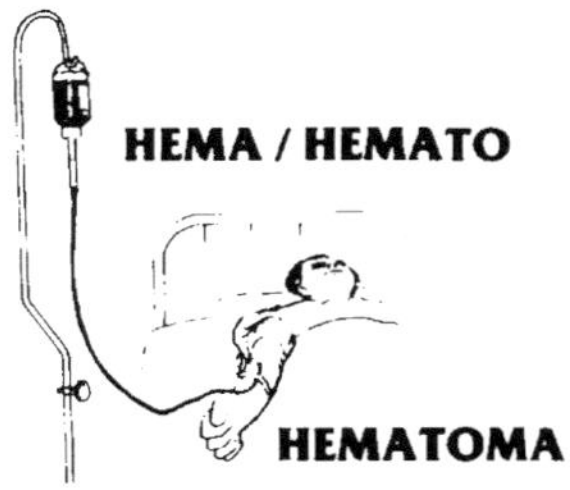

hem"ah-to'mah

blood

****

83. Lympho is a stem which means lymph. A lymphocyte is a _________ cell.

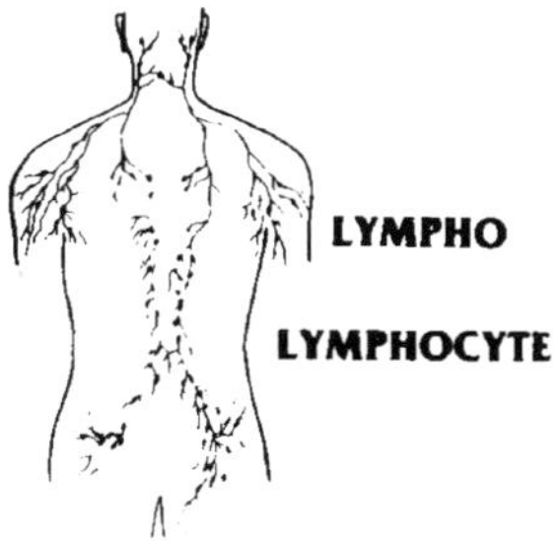

lim'fo-sit

lymph

****

84. Spleno is a stem which means spleen. A person who has had a splenectomy has had an excision of the __________.

sple-nek'to-me

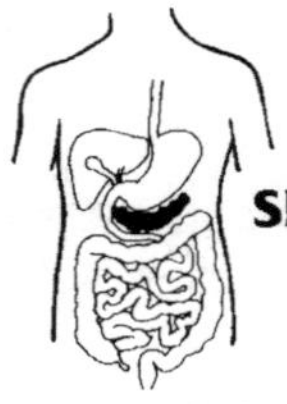

spleen

****

85. Phago is a stem which means to eat. A phagocyte is a cell that _________ microorganisms.

fag'o-sit

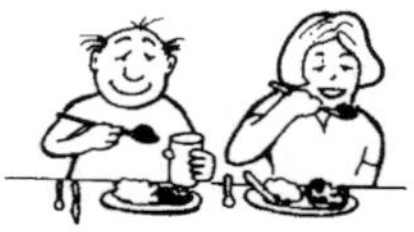

eats

****

86. As a review, give the meaning of each of the following stems pertaining to the hematopoietic and lymphatic systems.

a. cyto: __________

cell (frame 81)

****

b. hema/hemato: __________

blood (frame 82)

****

c. Spleno: __________

spleen (frame 84)

****

d. lympho: __________

lymph (frame 83)

****

e. phago: __________

to eat (frame 85)

****

87. To further reinforce what you have learned, fill in the blanks with the appropriate terms:

a. Cytology is the study of __________.

cells (frame 81)

****

b. Hematology is the study of __________.

hem'ah tol'o-je

blood (frame 82)

****

c. A lymphocyte is a __________ cell.

lymph (frame 83)

****

d. Splenectomy means excising of the __________.

spleen (frame 84)

****

e. Polyphagia means excessive __________.

pol"e-fa'je-ah

eating (frame 85)

****

If you missed any of the questions in frames 86 and 87, please review the appropriate frame(s) before continuing to frame 88.

Section X. STEMS - PERTAINING TO THE ENDOCRINE SYSTEM

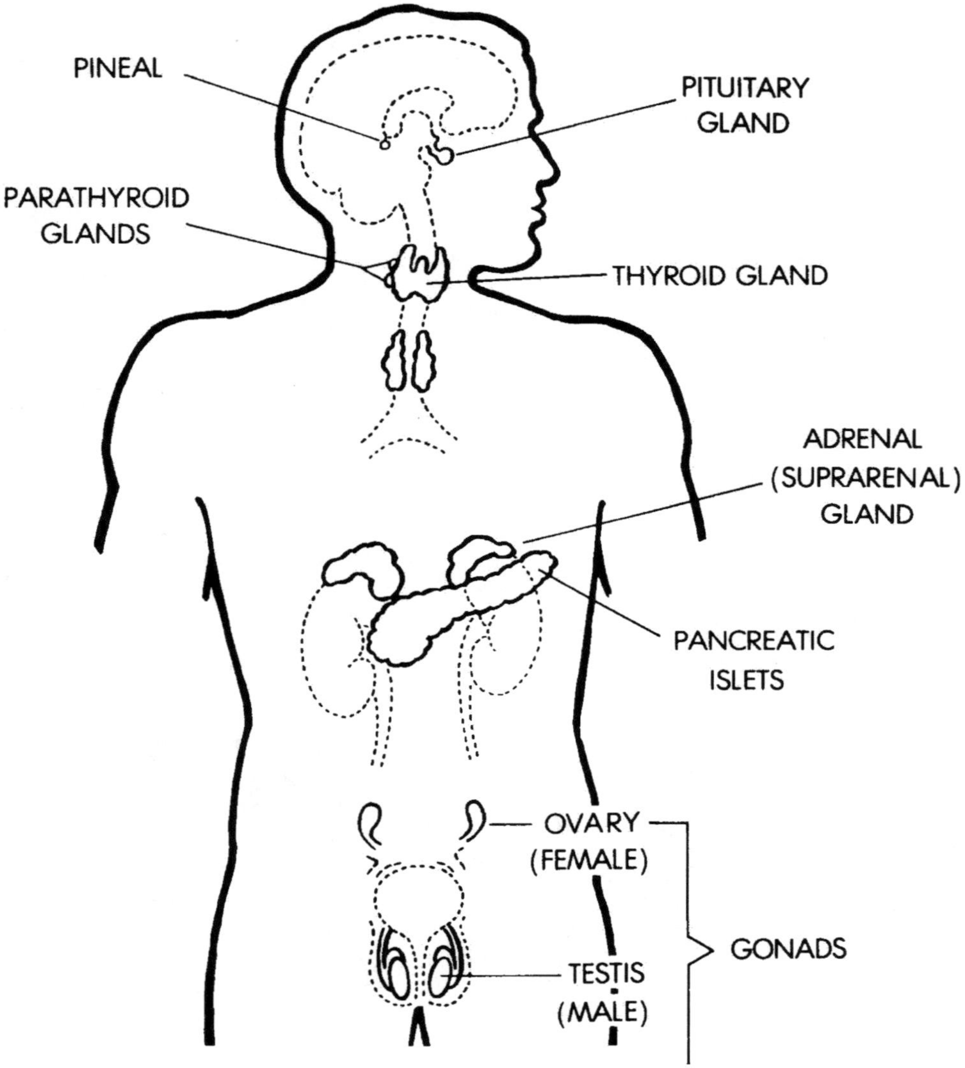

The endocrine system is composed of glands which release hormones into the blood stream.

****

88. Acro is a stem which means extremity. Acromegaly is a disease characterized by enlargement of the bones of the __________.

ak"ro meg' ah-le

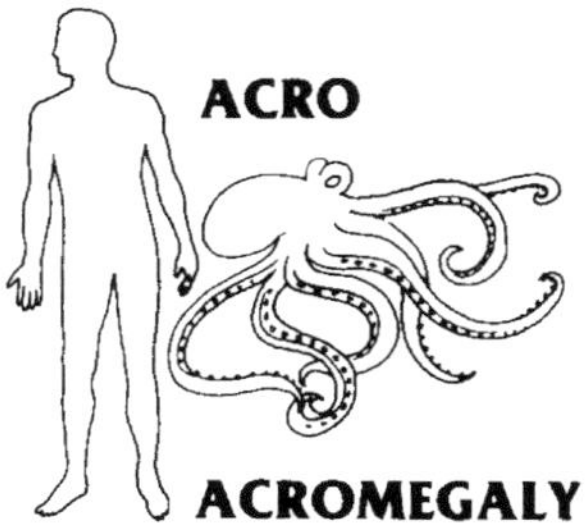

extremities

****

89. Gluco and glyco are stems which mean sugar. A person with glucosuria has __________ in the urine.

gloo"ko-su're-ah

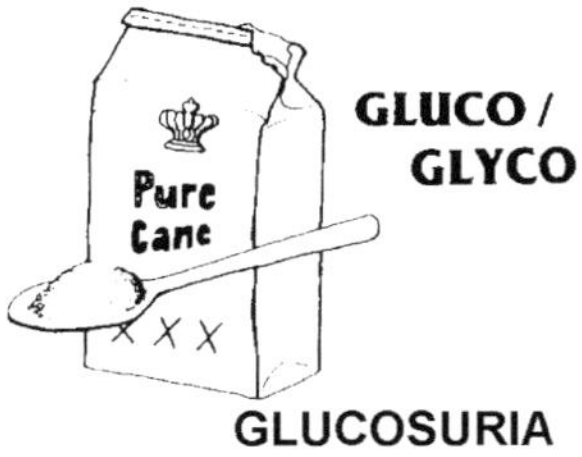

sugar

****

90. Adeno is a stem which means gland. Adenectomy is a word meaning surgical removal of a __________.

ad"e-nek' to-me

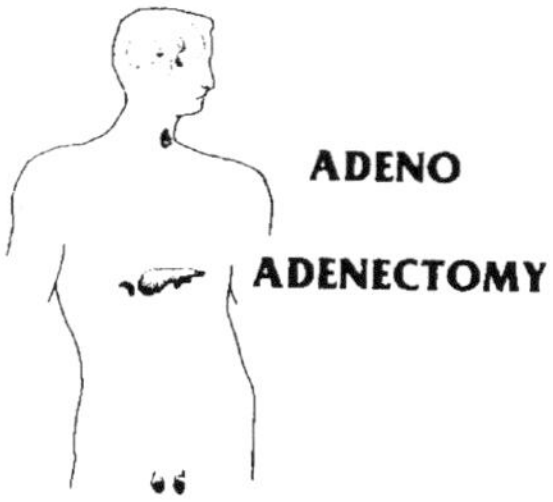

gland

****

91. As a review, give the meaning of the following stems:

a. acro: __________

extremity (frame 88)

****

b. gluco/glyco: __________

sugar (frame 89)

****

c. adeno: __________

gland (frame 90)

****

92. To further reinforce what you have learned, fill in the blank with the appropriate terms:

a. Acrodermatitis is a word that means inflammation of the skin of the __________.

ak"ro-der"mah-ti'tis

extremities (frame 88)

****

b. A person with glucosuria has __________in the urine.

sugar (frame 89)

****

c. A person who has had an adenectomy has had surgical removal of a __________.

gland (frame 90)

****

If you missed any of the questions in frames 91 and 92, please review the appropriate frame(s) before continuing to frame 93.

Section XI. STEMS - PERTAINING TO THE NERVOUS SYSTEM AND PSYCHIATRIC DISORDERS

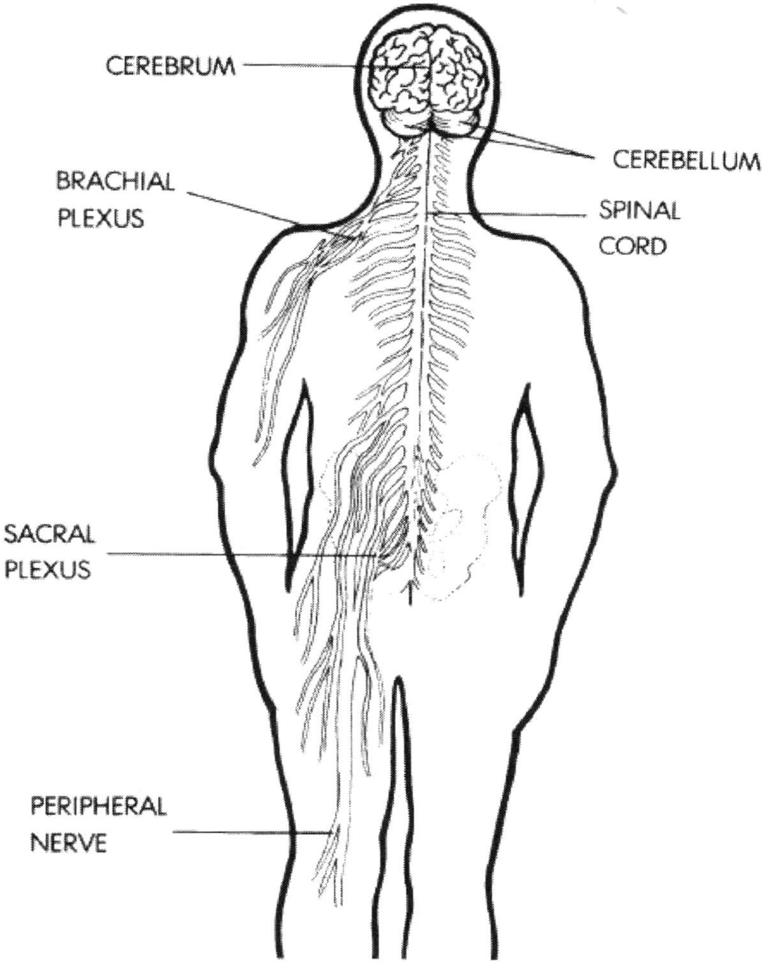

The nervous system along with the endocrine system correlates our adjustments and reactions to internal and environmental conditions.

****

93. Neuro is a stem which means nerve. Polyneuritis means inflammation of many __________.

pol"e-nu-ri'tis

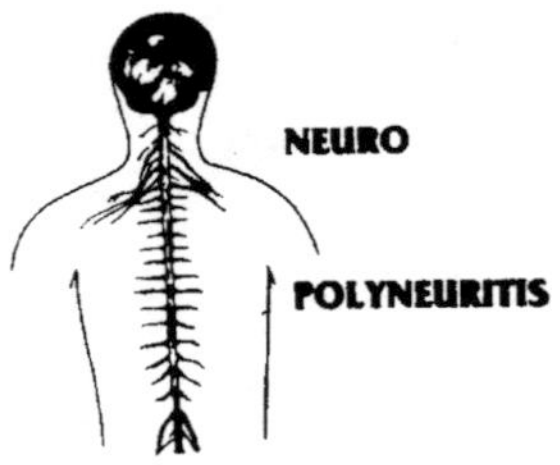

nerves

****

94. Cerebro and encephalo are stems which mean brain. Encephalitis, for example, means inflammation of the __________.

en"sef-ah-li'tis

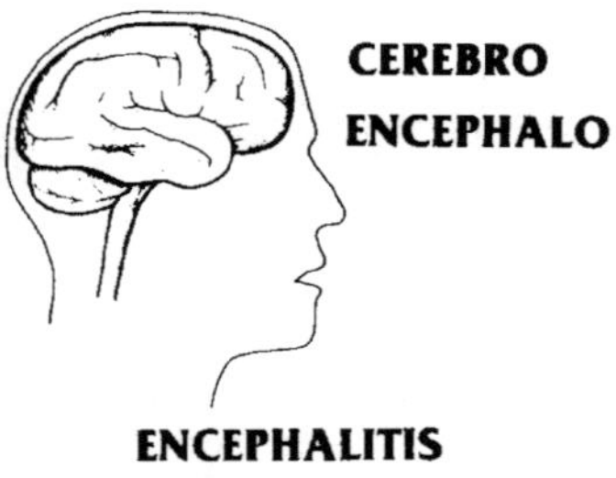

brain

****

95. Psycho and mento are stems which mean mind. Psychology is the science that studies the __________.

si-kol 'o-je

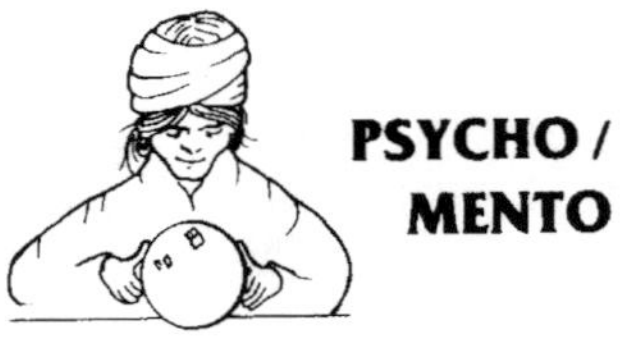

mind

****

96. Mania is a stem which means madness. Pyromania, for example, means fire __________.

pi"ro-ma'ne-ah

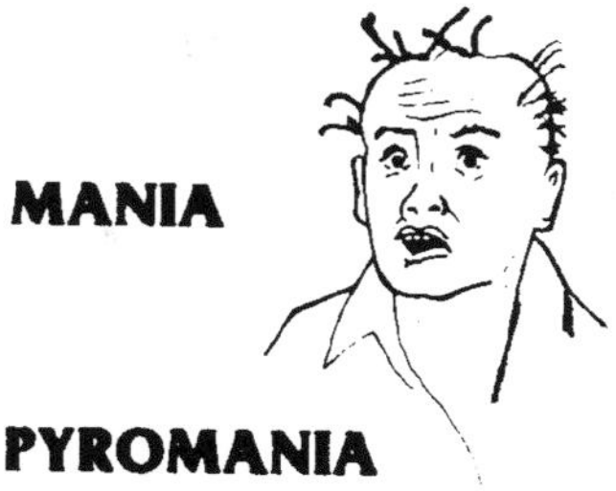

madness

****

97. Phobia is a stem which means fear. A person with hydrophobia has a __________ of water.

hi"dro-fo'be-ah

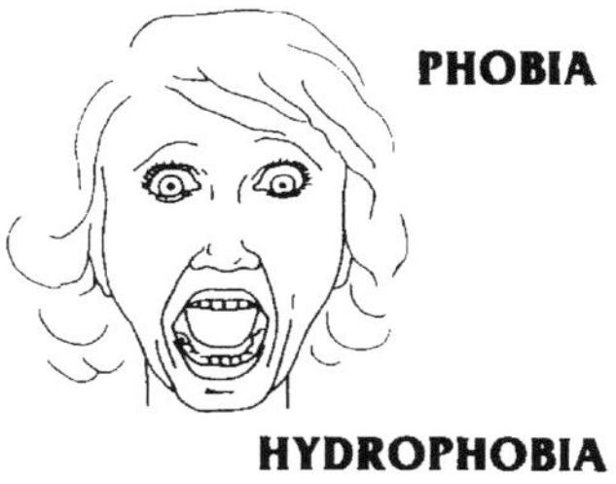

fear

****

98. Esthesia is a stem which means feeling or sensation. Anesthesia means without __________ or __________.

an"es-the'ze-ah

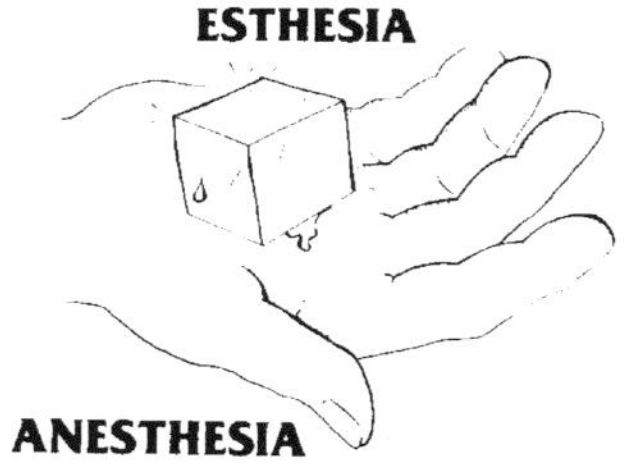

feeling/sensation

****

99. As a review, give the meaning of the following terms:

a. neuro: __________

nerve (frame 93)

****

b. cerebro/enchephalo: __________

brain (frame 94)

****

c. psycho/mento: __________

mind (frame 95)

****

d. mania: __________

madness (frame 96)

****

e. phobia: __________

fear (frame 97)

****

f. esthesia: __________

feeling/sensation (frame 98)

****

100 To further reinforce what you have learned, fill in the blanks with the appropriate terms:

a. Polyneuritis is an inflammation of many __________.

nerves (frame 93)

****

b. Encephalitis is an inflammation of the __________.

brain (frame 94)

****

c. Psychology is the science that studies the __________.

mind (frame 95)

****

d. Pyromania means fire __________.

madness (frame 96)

****

e. A person with hydrophobia has a __________ of water.

fear (frame 97)

****

f. Anesthesia means without

___________.

feeling/sensation (frame 98)

****

If you missed any of the questions in frames 99 and 100, please review the appropriate frame(s) before continuing to frame 101.

Section XII. STEMS - PERTAINING TO THE GENITOURINARY SYSTEM

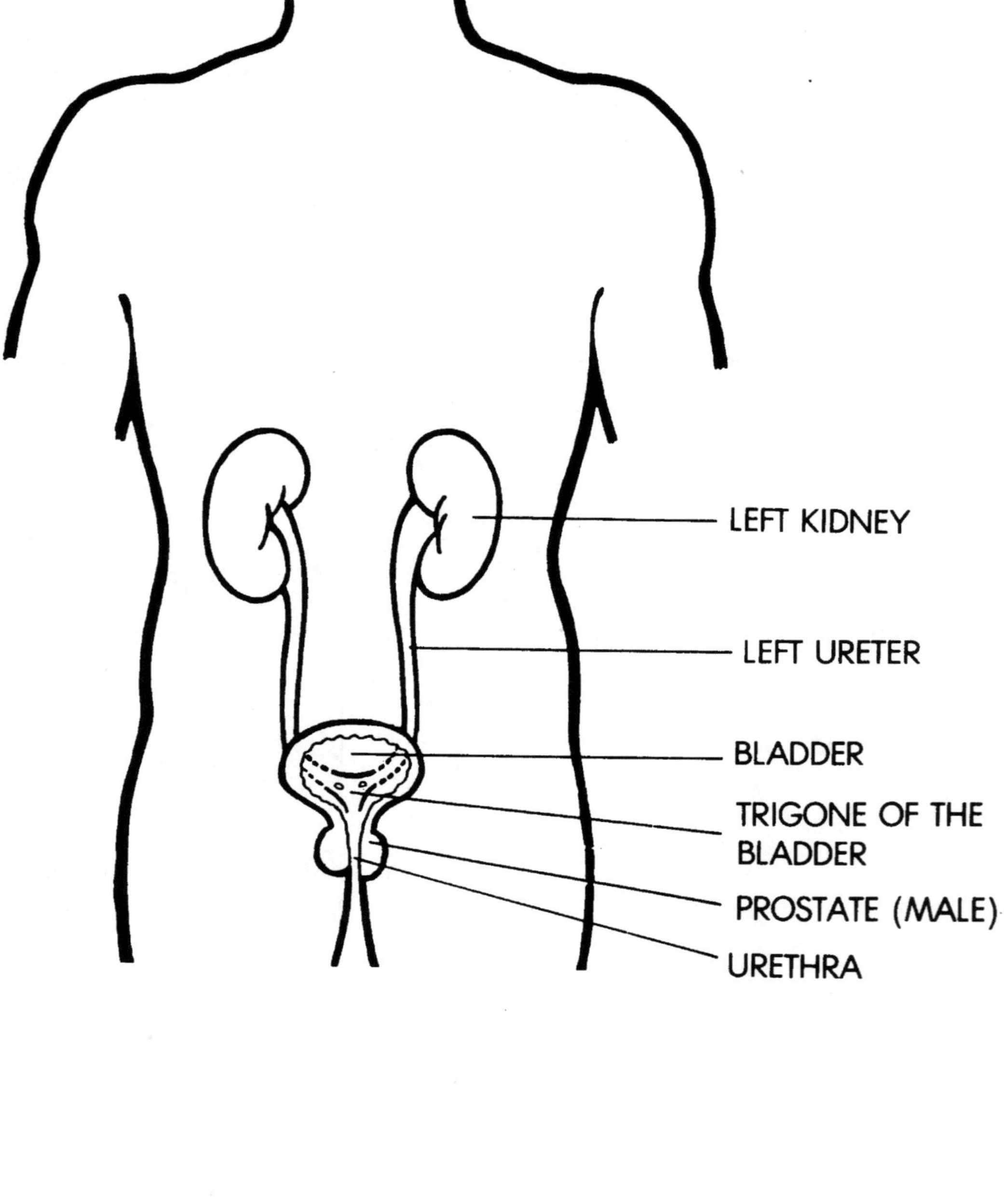

The genitourinary system includes the genitals and the urinary organs.

****

101 Nephro and rena are stems which mean kidney. A person who has had a nephrectomy has had a __________ removed.

ne-frek'to-m

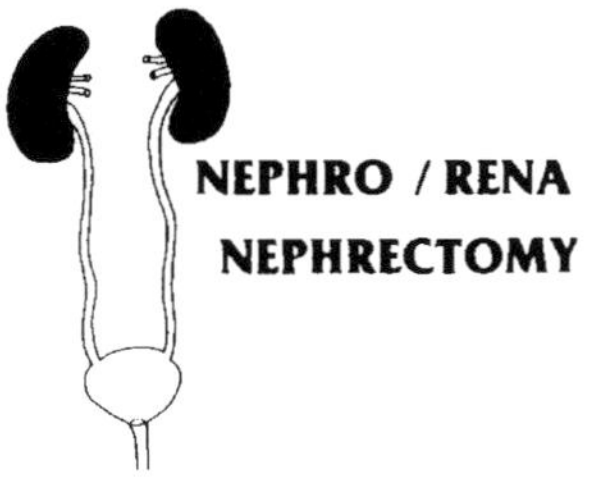

kidney

****

102 Uretero is a stem which means ureter. A person who has ureteritis has an inflammation of the __________.

u"re-ter-i'tis

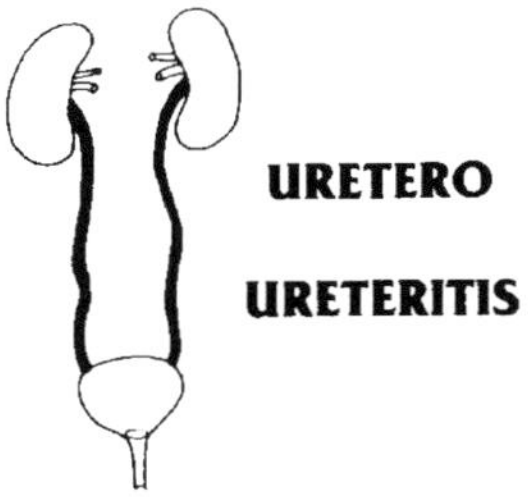

ureter

****

103 Cysto is a stem which means bladder. A person who has cystitis has an inflammation of the __________.

sis-ti-tis

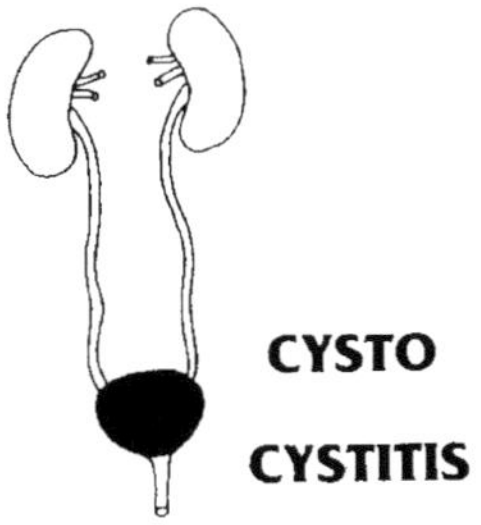

bladder

****

104 Urethro is a stem meaning urethra. Urethritis is an inflammation of the .

u"re-thri'tis

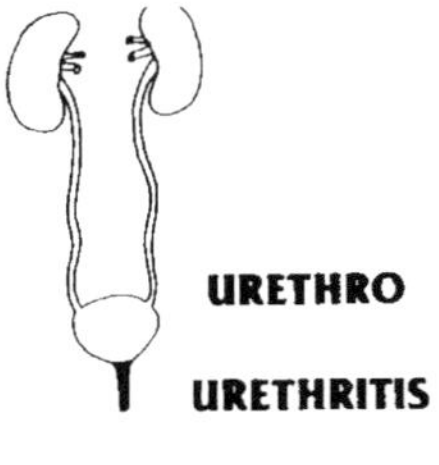

urethra

****

105 Orchio is a stem which means testes. Orchiopexy means fixation of the ___________.

or"ke-o-pek'se

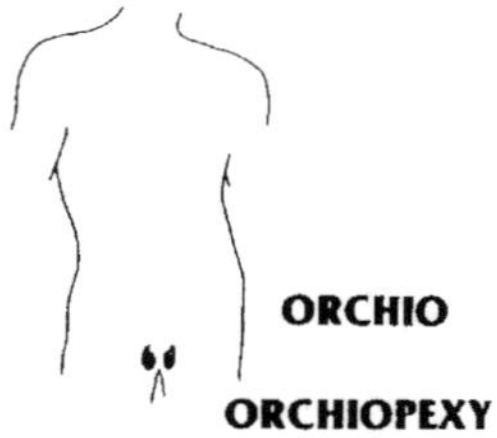

testes

****

106 Uro and uria are stems which mean urine. Urophobia is a term which means fear of passing __________.

u"ro-fo'be-ah

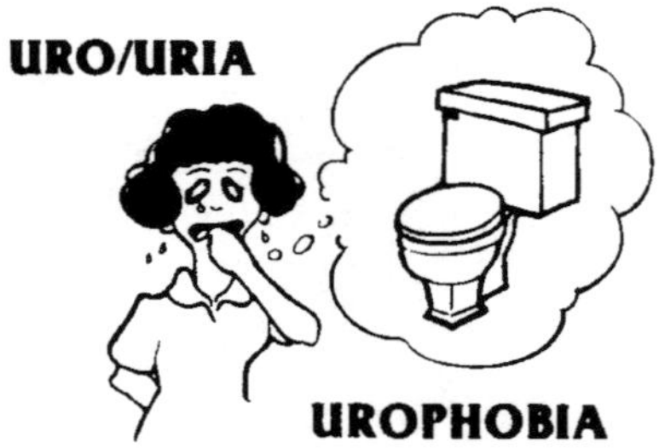

urine

****

107 Lith is a stem which means stone. Nephrolithiasis is the formation of renal __________.

nef"ro-li-thi'ah-sis

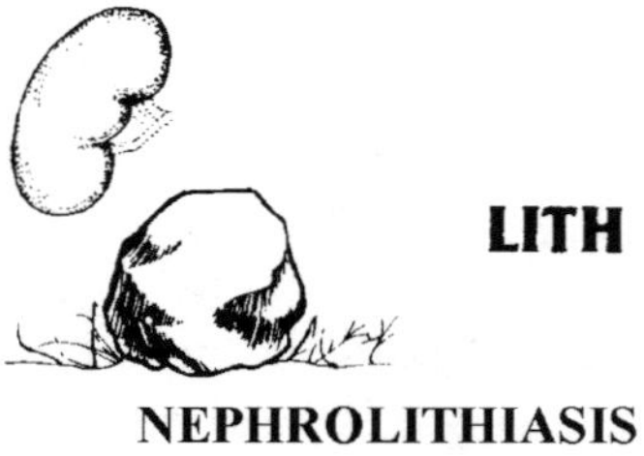

stones

****

108 In review, give the meaning of each of the following terms:

a. nephro/reno: __________

kidney (frame 101)

****

b. uretero: __________

ureter (frame 102)

****

c. cysto: __________

bladder (frame 103)

****

d. urethro: __________

urethra (frame 104)

****

e. orchio: ___________

testes (frame 105)

****

f. uro/uria: __________

urine (frame 106)

****

g. lith: __________

stone (frame 107)

****

109 To further reinforce what you have learned, fill in the blanks with the appropriate terms:

a. A person who has had a nephrectomy has had a __________ removed.

kidney (frame 101)

****

b. A person who has ureteritis has an inflammation of the __________.

ureter (frame 102)

****

c. Someone who has cystitis has an inflammation of the __________.

bladder (frame 103)

****

d. Urethritis is an inflammation of the __________.

urethra (frame 104)

****

e. Orchiopexy is the fixation of the
__________.

testes (frame 105)

****

f. Nephrolithiasis is the formation of renal __________.

stones (frame 107)

****

If you missed any of the questions in frames 108 and 109, please review the appropriate frame(s) before continuing to frame 110.

Section XIII. STEMS - PERTAINING TO GYNECOLOGY AND OBSTETRICS

FEMALE REPRODUCTIVE SYSTEM

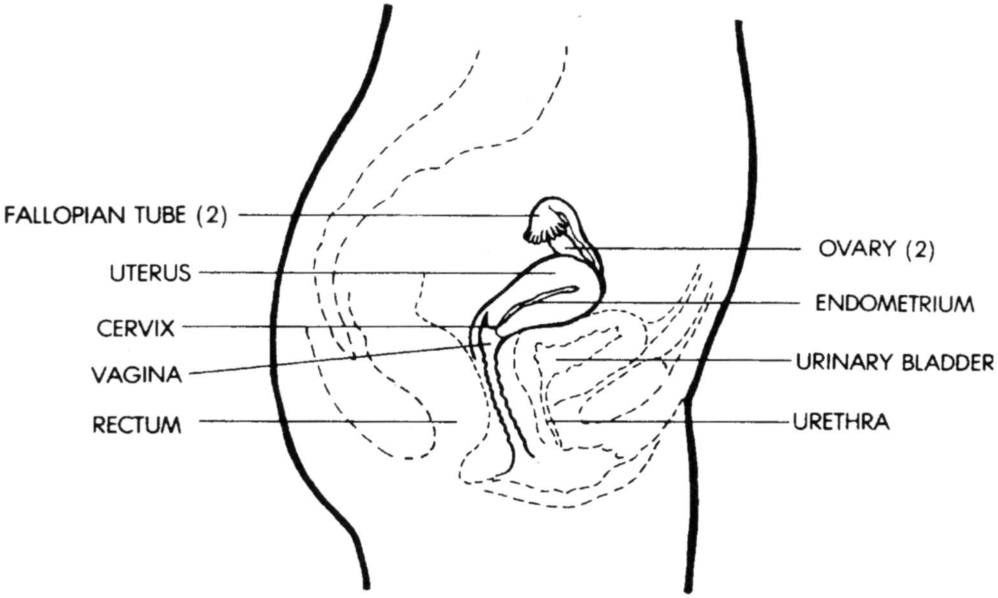

Gynecology and obstetrics relates to the female reproductive system and birth.

****

110 Hystero and metro are stems which mean uterus or womb. A woman who has had a hysterectomy, for example, has had her __________ removed.

his"te-rek'to-me

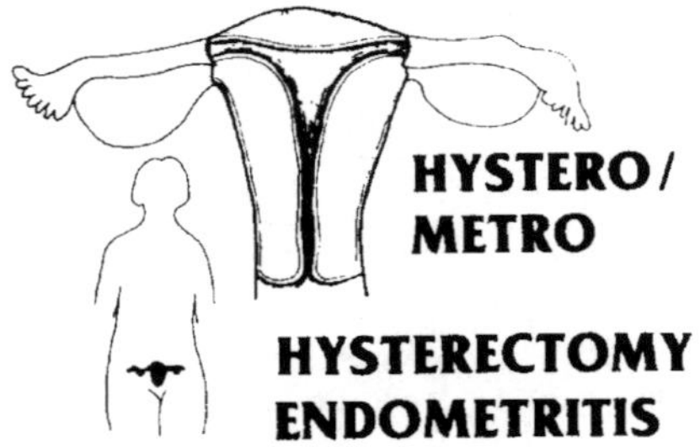

uterus

****

111 Oophoro is a stem which means ovary. A woman who has had an oophorectomy has had her __________ removed.

o"of-o-rek'to-me

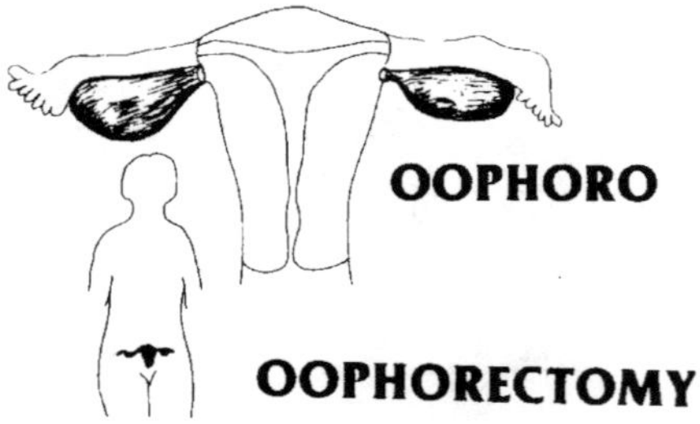

ovary

****

112 Salpingo is a stem which means tube. A woman who has salpingitis has an inflammation of a __________.

sal"pin-ji'tis

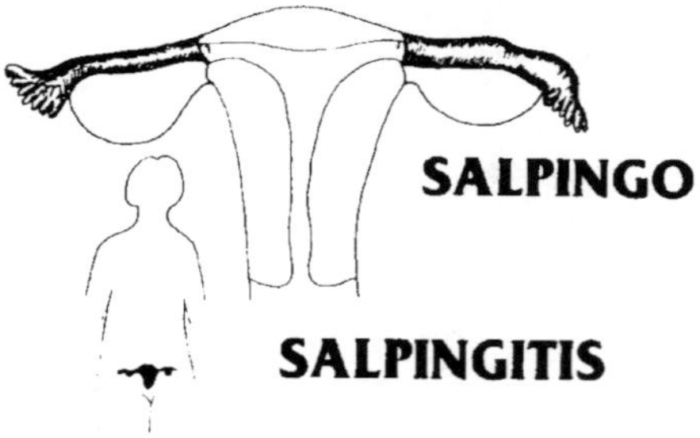

tube

****

113 As a review, give the meaning of each of the following terms:

a. hystero/metro: __________

uterus/womb (frame 110)

****

b. oophoro: __________

ovary (frame 111)

****

c. salpingo: __________

tube (frame 112)

****

114 To further reinforce what you have learned, fill in the blanks with the appropriate terms:

a. A woman who has had a hysterectomy has had her __________ removed.

uterus (frame 110)

****

b. When a woman has an oophorectomy, she has an __________ removed.

ovary (frame 111)

****

c. A woman who has salpingitis has an inflammation of the __________.

tube (frame 112)

****

If you missed any of the questions in frames 113 and 114, please review the appropriate frame(s) before continuing to frame 115.

Section XIV. STEMS - PERTAINING TO THE SENSORY ORGANS

SENSORY ORGANS

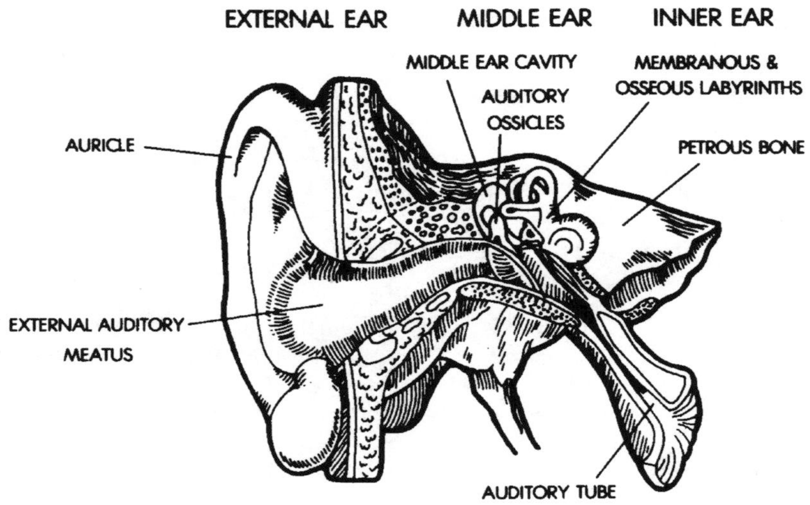

SENSORY ORGANS

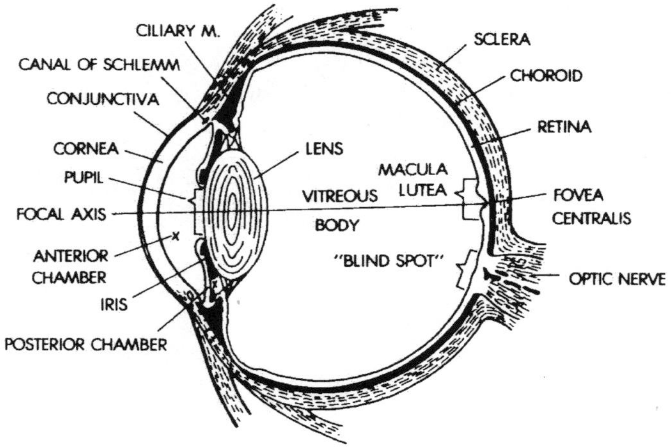

The sensory organs, as you know, include the eye and the ear.

****

115 Oto is a stem which means ear. Otoplasty, for example, means plastic repair of the __________.

o'to-plas"te

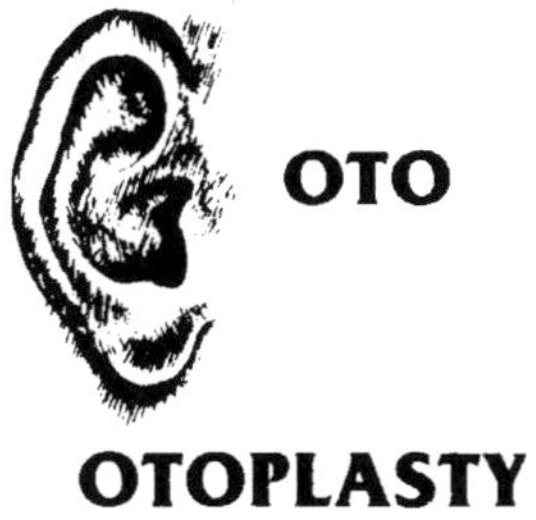

ear

****

116 Tympano and myringo are stems which refer to the eardrum. A tympanoplasty means plastic repair of the __________.

tim"pah-no-plas'te

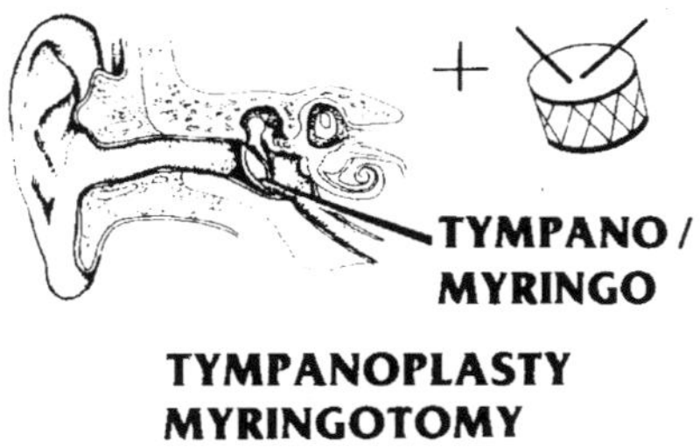

eardrum

****

117 Ophthalmo and oculo are stems which mean eye. Ophthalmology is the science dealing with the __________ and its diseases.

of"thal-mol'o-je

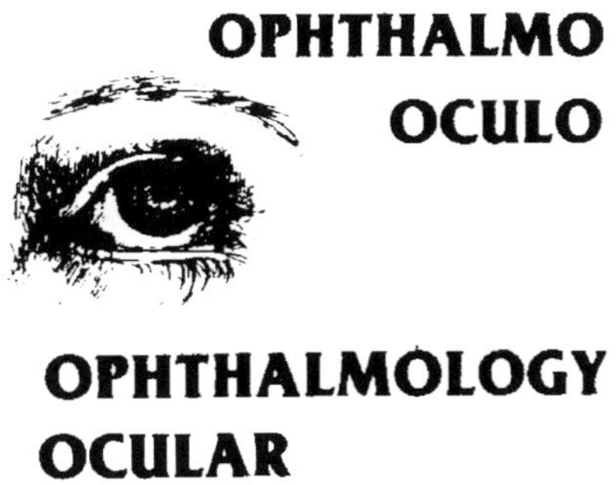

eye

****

118 Opto is a stem which means vision. An optometrist is a person who is trained to examine eyes in order to determine the presence of __________ problems.

op-tom'e-trist

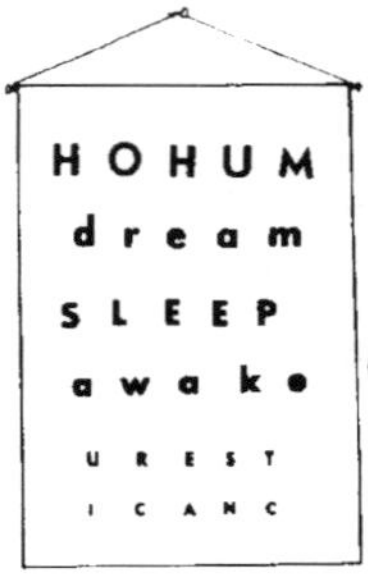

OPTO

OPTOMETRIST

vision

****

119 Blepharo is a stem which means eyelid. Blepharitis means inflammation of the __________.

blef"ah-ri'tis

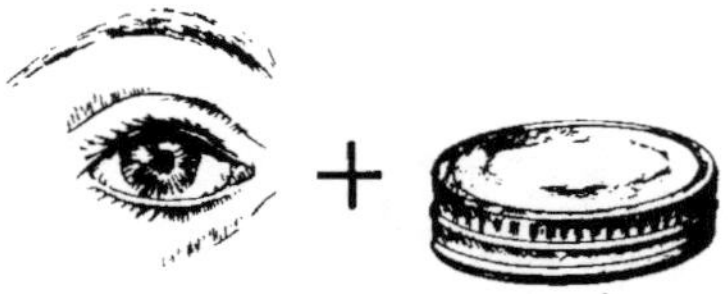

BLEPHARO

BLEPHARITIS

eyelid

****

120 Kerato is a stem which means cornea. Keratitis means inflammation of the __________.

ker"ah-ti'tis

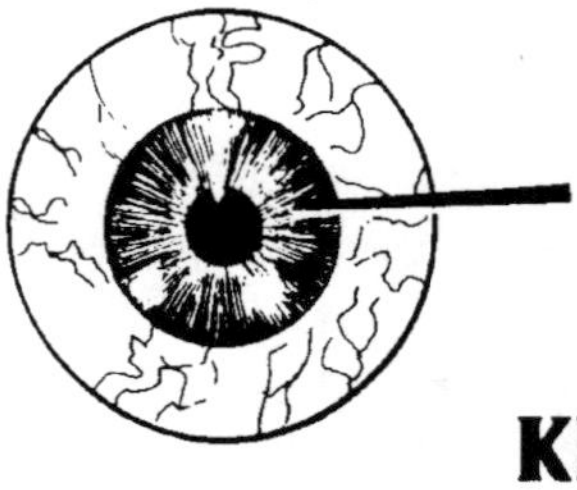

KERATO

KERATITIS

cornea

****

121 Dacryo is a stem which means tear. A person with dacryocystitis has inflammation of the __________ sac.

dak"re-o-sis-ti'tis

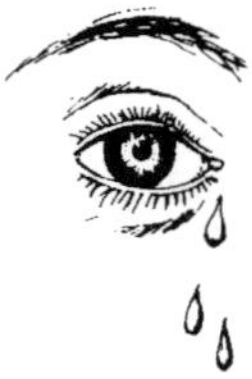

DACRYO

DACRYOCYSTITIS

tear

****

122 As a review, give the meaning of each of the following terms:

a. oto: __________

ear (frame 115)

****

b. tympano/myringo: __________

eardrum (frame 116)

****

c. ophthalmo/oculo: __________

eye (frame 117)

****

d. opto: __________

vision (frame 118)

****

e. blepharo: __________

eyelid (frame 119)

****

f. kerato: __________

cornea (frame 120)

****

g. dacryo: __________

tear (frame 121)

****

123 To further reinforce what you have learned, fill in the blanks with the appropriate terms:

a. Otoplasty is the plastic repair of the __________.

ear (frame 115)

****

b. A tympanoplasty is the plastic repair of the __________.

eardrum (frame 116)

****

c. Ophthalmology is the science dealing with the __________ and its diseases.

eye (frame 117)

****

d. An optometrist is a person who is trained to examine eyes in order to determine the presence of __________ problems.

vision (frame 118)

****

e. Blepharitis is an inflammation of the __________.

eyelid (frame 119)

****

f. Keratitis is an inflammation of the __________.

cornea (frame 120)

****

g. A person with dacryocysitis has an inflammation of the __________ sac.

tear (frame 121)

****

If you missed any of the questions in frames 122 and 123, please review the appropriate frame(s) before continuing to frame 124.

EMESIS-

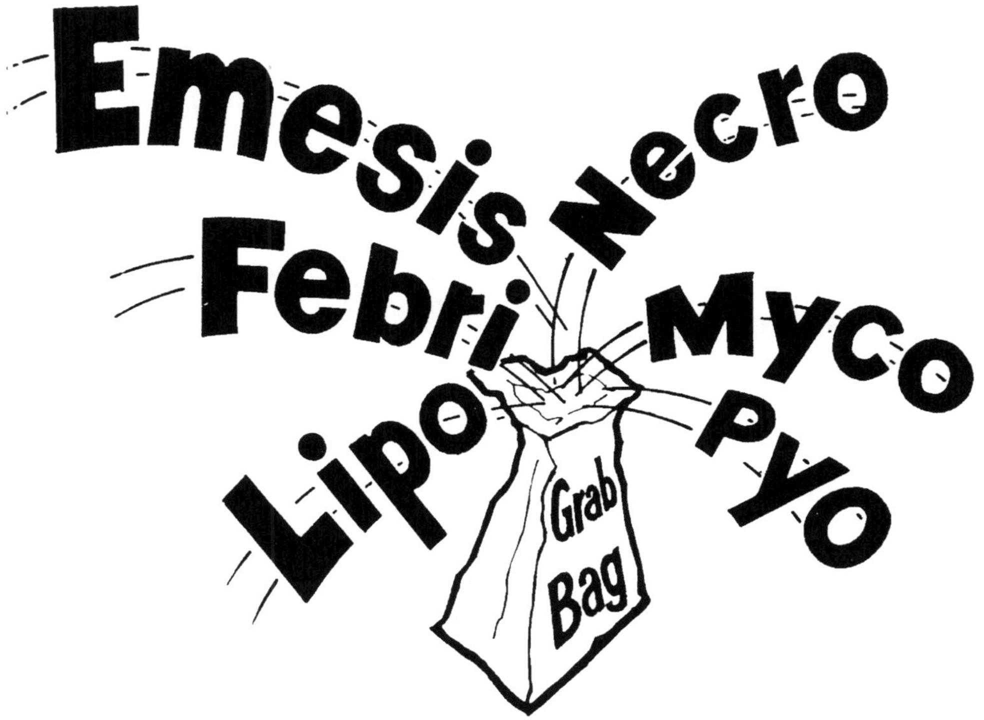

****

124 Pyo is a stem meaning pus. The word pyogenic means producing __________.

pi"o-jen'ik

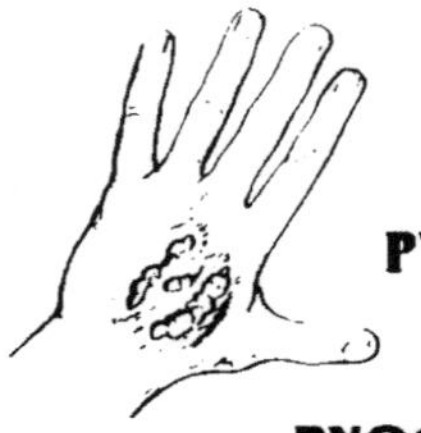

pus

****

125 Lipo is a stem which means fat. A lipoma is a tumor composed of __________.

li-po mah

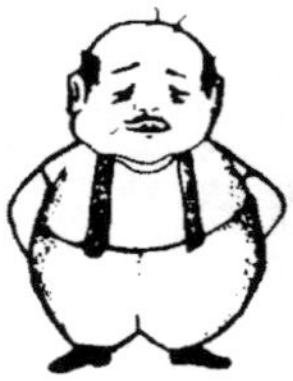

fat

****

126 Febri is a stem which means fever. A person who is afebrile is without __________.

a-feb'ril

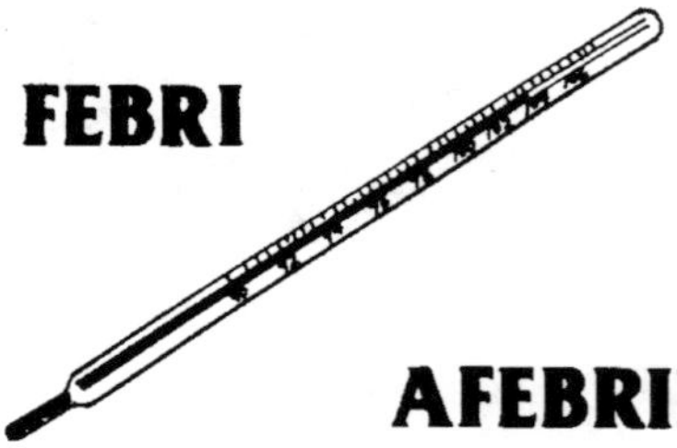

fever

****

127 Myco is a stem which means fungus. Mycosis is any disease caused by a __________.

mi-ko'sis

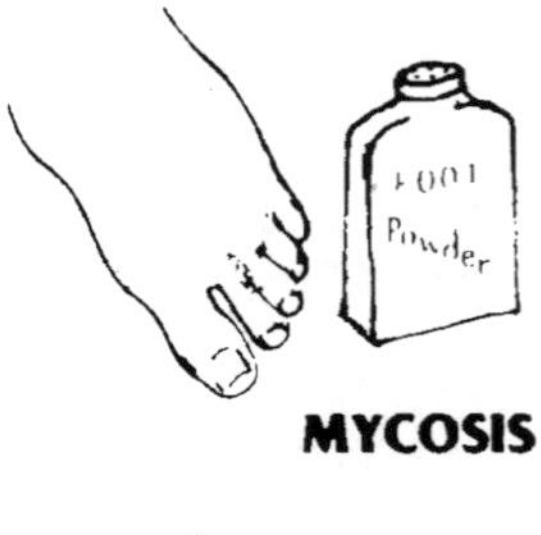

fungus

****

128 Necro is a stem which means dead. A necropsy is an autopsy or scientific inspection of a __________ body.

nek'rop-se

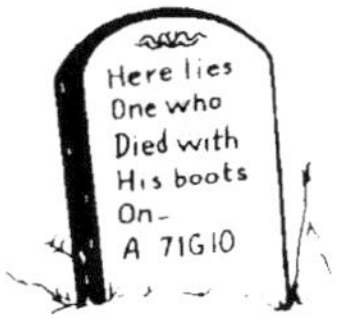

NECRO

NECROPSY

dead

****

129 Emesis is a stem which means vomit. Hyperemesis is a word which means excessive __________.

hi"per-em'e-sis

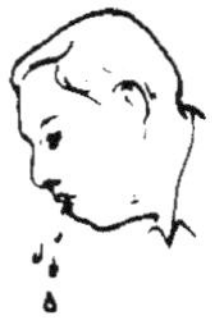

EMESIS

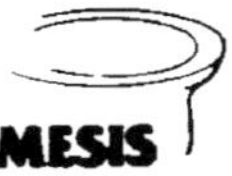

HYPEREMESIS

vomiting

****

130 As a review, give the meaning of each of the following terms:

a. pyo: __________

pus (frame 124)

****

b. lipo: __________

fat (frame 125)

****

c. febri: __________

fever (frame 126)

****

d. myco: __________

fungus (frame 127)

****

e. necro: __________

dead (frame 128)

****

f. emesis: __________

vomiting (frame 129)

****

131 To further reinforce what you have learned, fill in the blanks with the appropriate words:

a. The term pyogenic means producing __________.

pus (frame 124)

****

b. A lipoma is a tumor composed of __________.

fat (frame 125)

****

c. A person who is afebrile is without __________.

fever (frame 126)

****

d. Mycosis is any disease caused by a __________.

fungus (frame 127)

****

e. A necropsy is an autopsy or scientific inspection of a __________ body.

dead (frame 128)

****

f. Hyperemesis is excessive __________.

vomiting (frame 129)

****

If you missed any of the questions in frames 130 and 131, please review the appropriate frame(s) before continuing.

You have now completed the first part of this programmed text on medical terminology.

Congratulations!

As a fun review and exercise, you can complete the stem crossword puzzle on the following page before completing the self-assessment questions starting on page 2-71.

Continue with Self-Assessment

Section XVI. MEDICAL TERMINOLOGY CROSSWORD PUZZLE

Fill in the combining forms for the stems listed below the puzzle.

Solutions are on page 2-78.

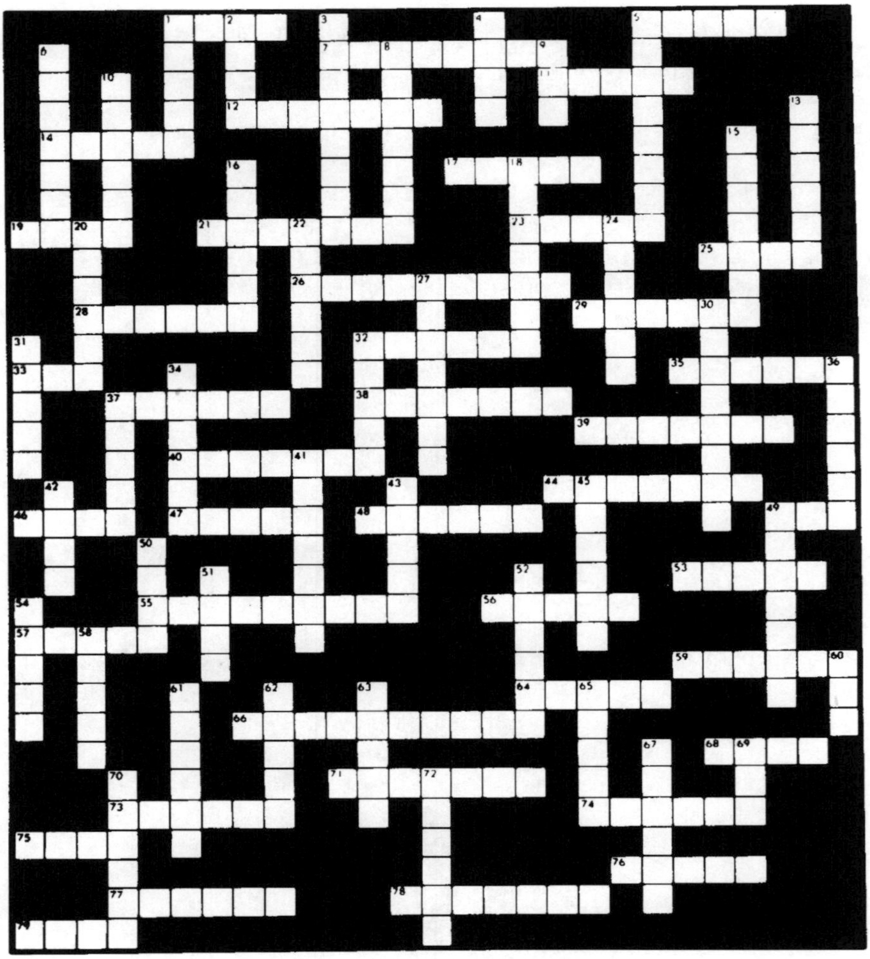

DOWN

1. MADNESS
2. CELL
3. FEELING
4. BREATH
5. ABDOMEN
6. DUODENUM
8. LARYNX
9. EAR
10. CORNEA
13. LIP
15. GUMS
16. MIND
18. CLOT
20. ABDOMINAL WALL
22. FEAR
24. KIDNEY
27. UTERUS
30. EYELID
31. LUNGS
32. SUGAR
34. RECTUM
36. NAILS
37. RIBS
41. BRONCHUS
42. VESSEL
43. GLAND
45. BLOOD
49. EARDRUM
50. ILEUM
51. EXTREMITY
52. JEJUNUM
54. EYE
58. MOUTH
60. ANUS
61. LUNGS
62. EATING
63. NERVE
65. ABDOMEN
67. TEARS
69. PUS
70. TONGUE
72. INTESTINE

ACROSS

1. FUNGUS
5. VESSEL
7. TUBE
11. TENDON
12. OVARY
14. SKIN
17. UTERUS
19. COLON
21. EARDRUM
23. NOSE
25. FAT
26. EYE
28. JOINT
29. VEIN
32. STOMACH
33. URINE
35. LIVER
37. HEART
38. URETHRA
39. TRACHEA
40. BRAIN
44. CARTILAGE
46. NOSE
47. BONE
48. TEETH
49. MUSCLE
53. FEVER
55. BRAIN
56. TOOTH
57. BLADDER
59. TONGUE
64. DEAD
66. GALL BLADDER
68. VISION
71. ARTERY
73. LYMPH
74. TESTES
75. VEIN
76. SPINAL CORD
77. SPLEEN
78. URETER
79. BLOOD

Section XVII. SELF-ASSESSMENT #1

To evaluate how well you have learned the stems covered in lesson 2, complete the self-assessment #1 questions. This self-assessment is to assist you in determining whether you need to go back and review parts of lesson 2 before going to lesson 3. The answers to the questions are given on pages 2-75 and 2-76.

SELF-ASSESSMENT #1

Stems

LISTED BELOW IN COLUMN "A" ARE 15 OF THE 100 LATIN AND GREEK STEMS GIVEN TO YOU. IN COLUMN "B" ARE THE ENGLISH MEANINGS OF THE STEMS. MATCH THE TWO, AND WRITE THE ENGLISH MEANING FROM COLUMN "B" IN COLUMN "A."

EXAMPLE: GLAND ADENO

COLUMN A			COLUMN B	
1.	______________	OSTEO	A.	URINE
2.	______________	ARTHRO	B.	BLOOD
3.	______________	CARDIO	C.	CELL
4.	______________	URO/URIA	D.	RIB
5.	______________	LIPO	E.	TONGUE
6.	______________	HEMO/HEMATO	F.	GALLBLADDER
7.	______________	THROMBO	G.	BONE
8.	______________	CYTO	H.	KIDNEY
9.	______________	COSTO	I.	NERVE
10.	______________	LINGUA/GLOSSA	J.	STOMACH
11.	______________	CHOLECYSTO	K.	HEART
12.	______________	NEPHRO/RENA	L.	EXTREMITY
13.	______________	NEURO	M.	FAT
14.	______________	GASTRO	N.	CLOT
15.	______________	ACRO	O.	JOINT

SELF-ASSESSMENT QUIZ #1

STEMS

FOR EACH OF THE MULTIPLE CHOICE QUESTIONS BELOW, SELECT THE ONE MOST APPROPRIATE ANSWER. CIRCLE THE ANSWER.

16. THE STEM "CHONDRO" IN THE WORD CHONDRITIS MEANS:

    A. TENDON
    B. RIB
    C. CARTILAGE
    D. JOINT

17. THE STEM "MYO" IN THE WORD MYOPLASM MEANS:

    A. CARTILAGE
    B. MUSCLE
    C. BONE
    D. VEIN

18. THE STEM "HEPATO" IN THE WORD HEPATITIS MEANS:

    A. BLOOD
    B. LIVER
    C. KIDNEY
    D. NAIL

19. THE STEM "ADENO" IN THE WORD ADENECTOMY MEANS:

    A. BLADDER
    B. GALLBLADDER
    C. ABDOMINAL WALL
    D. GLAND

20. THE STEM "MYCO" IN THE WORD MYCOSIS MEANS:

    A. SKIN
    B. CELL
    C. CLOT
    D. FUNGUS

21. THE STEM "EMESIS" IN THE WORD HYPEREMESIS MEANS:

    A. SCANT
    B. EXCESSIVE
    C. VOMITING
    D. EXIT

22. THE STEM "FEBRI" IN THE WORD AFEBRILE MEANS:

    A. FEVER
    B. FUNGUS
    C. FAT
    D. FEELING

23. THE STEM "ENCEPHALO" IN THE WORD ENCEPHALITIS MEANS:

A. BRAIN
B. HEAD
C. SPINE
D. TOOTH

24. THE STEM "ARTERIO" IN THE WORD ARTERIOSCLEROSIS MEANS:

A. VEIN
B. ARTERY
C. JOINT
D. CARTILAGE

25. THE STEM "LAPARO" IN THE WORD LAPARATOMY MEANS:

A. ABDOMINAL WALL
B. CELL WALL
C. URINARY BLADDER
D. STOMACH

Check your answers on the following pages

SOLUTIONS FOR SELF-ASSESSMENT #1

<u>Stems</u>

1. G (BONE) OSTEO
2. O (JOINT) ARTHRO
3. K (HEART) CARDIO
4. A (URINE) URO/URIA
5. M (FAT) LIPO
6. B (BLOOD) HEMO/HEMATO
7. N (CLOT) THROMBO
8. C (CELL) CYTO
9. D (RIB) COSTO
10. E (TONGUE) LINGUA/GLOSSA
11. F (GALLBLADDER) CHOLECYSTO
12. H (KIDNEY) NEPHRO/RENA
13. I (NERVE) NEURO
14. J (STOMACH) GASTRO
15. L (EXTREMITY) ACRO

SOLUTIONS FOR SELF-ASSESSMENTQUIZ #1

Stems

16. THE STEM "CHONDRO" IN THE WORD CHONDRITIS MEANS:

C. CARTILAGE

17. THE STEM "MYO" IN THE WORD MYOPLASM MEANS:

B. MUSCLE

18. THE STEM "HEPATO" IN THE WORD HEPATITIS MEANS:

B. LIVER

19. THE STEM "ADENO" IN THE WORD ADENECTOMY MEANS:

D. GLAND

20. THE STEM "MYCO" IN THE WORD MYCOSIS MEANS:

D. FUNGUS

21. THE STEM "EMESIS" IN THE WORD HYPEREMESIS MEANS:

C. VOMITING

22. THE STEM "FEBRI" IN THE WORD AFEBRILE MEANS:

A. FEVER

23. THE STEM "ENCEPHALO" IN THE WORD ENCEPHALITIS MEANS:

A. BRAIN

24. THE STEM "ARTERIO" IN THE WORD ARTERIOSCLEROSIS MEANS:

B. ARTERY

25. THE STEM "LAPARO" IN THE WORD LAPARATOMY MEANS:

A. ABDOMINAL WALL

SOLUTIONS TO PRETEST #1

1. eye
2. ear
3. birth/fever
4. tube
5. ovary
6. stone
7. urine
8. testicle
9. bladder
10. urethra
11. gall
12. uterus, tubes, and ovaries
13. herniation
14. feeling/sensation
15. fear
16. disorder
17. bone
18. brain (cerebrum)
19. nerve
20. sugar
21. swelling
22. extremities
23. eating
24. spleen
25. lymph
26. brain
27. fat
28. pus
29. tears
30. cells
31. clot
32. arteries
33. veins
34. vessel
35. vessel
36. liver
37. rectum/anus
38. colon
39. jejunum - ileum
40. mental
41. intestine
42. stomach
43. gums
44. tears
45. lips
46. duodenum
47. mouth
48. breathing
49. air
50. abdominal wall
51. tongue
52. bronchial
53. nose
54. nose
55. larynx
56. nails
57. ribs
58. abdomen
59. tendon
60. muscle
61. spinal cord
62. cartilage
63. joint
64. tympanic membrane
65. cornea
66. pharynx
67. eyelid
68. blood
69. dead
70. fungus

Go to Lesson 3

Continue with Lesson 2

SOLUTION TO MEDICAL TERMINOLOGY CROSSWORD PUZZLE

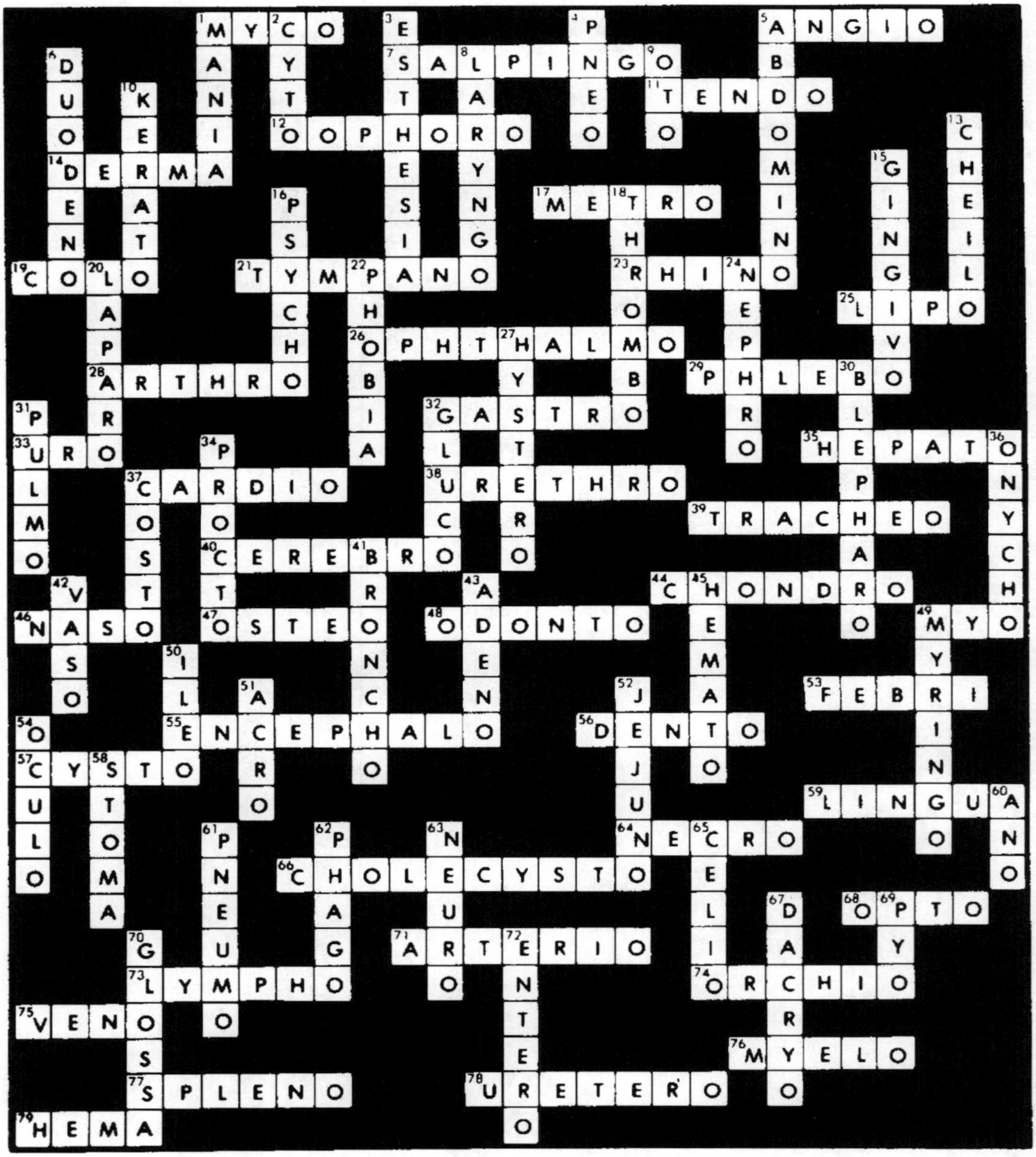

LESSON ASSIGNMENT

LESSON 3	Prefixes Pertaining to Medical Terminology.
LESSON ASSIGNMENT	Lesson 3, frame numbers 132-198.
LESSON OBJECTIVES	After completing this lesson, you should be able to:

3-1. Given 10 of the 50 Latin and Greek medical related prefixes and a list of English meanings for these prefixes, write the English meaning in the space provided without error.

3-2. Given 10 multiple choice questions on medical prefixes, select the most appropriate answer without error.

LESSON 3

Section I. PRETEST #2

Before you turn to frame 132 and begin work on your study of prefixes in medical terminology, complete pretest #2. The pretest contains 31 questions relating to medical terminology prefixes. If you correctly answer 90% or more of the questions, you pass the pretest. A score of 90% on this pretest is 27 correct answers.

Write your answers in the space provided in each question.

1. Malnutrition means ________________ nutrition.

2. Noctiphobia is an abnormal fear of ______________.

3. Dysmenorrhea means _______________ menstrual flow.

4. Hydrotherapy is treatment with ________________.

5. Macrorhinia means ____________________ nose.

6. A baby born with a microcephalus had a very _______ head.

7. A melanoma is a ___________________ tumor.

8. Cyanopia is a defect in vision that causes objects to appear _______________________________.

9. Erythroderma means ___________________ skin.

10. A leukoblast is a _______________ embryonic cell.

11. Oligopnea means __________________ breathing.

12. Bradypepsia means _________________ digestion.

13. Tachyphasia means ___________________ speech.

14. A monocyte has ___________________ cell(s).

15. Asepsia means ___________________ infection.

16. Hyperalgesia is _____________ sensitivity to pain.

17. Hemifacial means pertaining to one ________ of the face.

18. Polyarthritis means inflammation of __________ joints.

19. Ectogenous is something produced _________ an organism.

20. Pericolic is a word for ______________ the colon.

21. A medication administered hypoglossal is placed ________ the tongue.

22. Subaural means ___________________ the ear.

23. Postcibal means ___________________ meals.

24. Ectocytic means __________________ the cell.

25. An antiseptic is a drug that works _________ infection.

26. Endocranial means ________________ the cranium.

27. Retrosternal means _______________ the sternum.

28. Ante mortem is ____________________ death.

29. Preoperative is ___________________ surgery.

30. An interdental cavity is _____________ the teeth.

31. Bilateral means pertaining to ____________ side(s).

Check your answers on page 3-39

Section II. PREFIXES - GENERAL INFORMATION

Prefixes are one or more letters or syllables which come <u>before</u> the stem (at the beginning of a word) to explain or add meaning to the rest of the term.

****

132 A prefix comes __________ the stem.

before

****

133 In the term unforgettable, "forget" is the stem and "un" is the __________.

prefix

****

134 In the words implant, supplant, and transplant, the prefixes are ______, ______, and ______.

imp/sup/trans

****

135 You can change the meaning of a term by putting a prefix before the __________.

stem

****

136 Prefixes are the most frequently used elements in the formation of Greek and Latin words, but not every word contains a __________.

prefix

****

137 Prefixes may be divided into various categories of meaning depending on how they modify the stem, such as location, time, amount, color, negation, size, or position. Prefixes may be divided into various categories of __________.

meaning

****

138 To reinforce what you have learned, please write the correct word in each of the blanks in the following sentences.

a. A prefix comes __________ the stem.

before (frame 132)

****

b. In the term unforgettable, "forget" is the stem and "un" is the __________.

prefix (frame 133)

****

c. In the words implant, supplant, and transplant, the prefixes are _____, _____, and _____.

imp/sup/trans (frame 134)

****

d. You can change the meaning of a term by putting a prefix before the __________.

stem (frame 135)

****

e. Not every Greek or Latin word contains a __________.

prefix (frame 136)

****

f. Prefixes may be divided into various categories of __________.

meaning (frame 137)

****

If you missed any of the questions in frame 138, please review the appropriate frame(s) before continuing to frame 139.

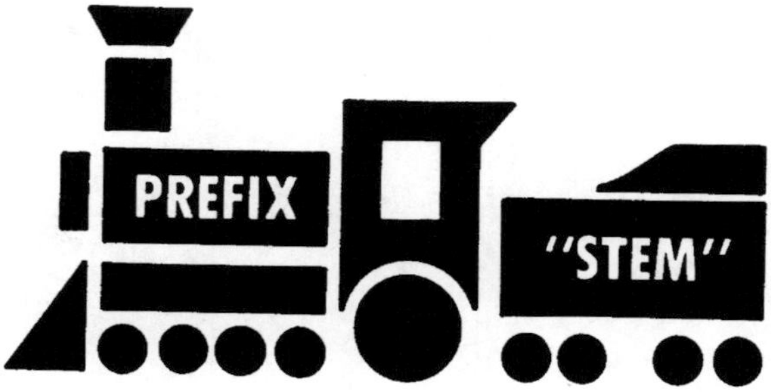

Section III. PREFIXES - PERTAINING TO LOCATION

We will now study the prefixes that indicate location.

****

139 The prefix intra- means inside or within. The dash after intra- indicates that the stem comes __________ (before, after) the prefix.

after

****

140 By combining the prefix intra- with the stem abdominal, you know it means __________ the abdomen.

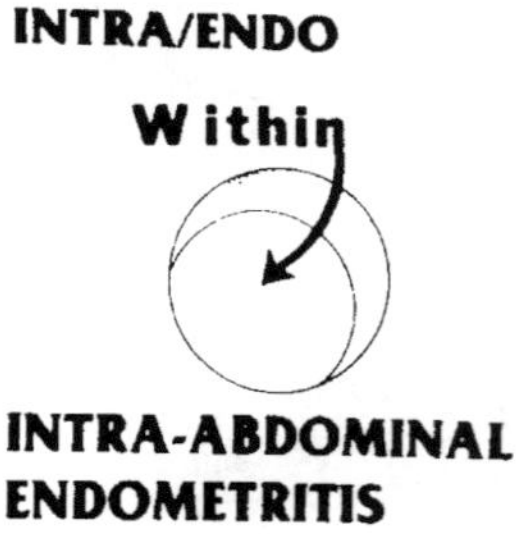

in"trah-ab-dom'i-nal

inside/within

****

141 Endo- is also a prefix meaning within or inside. Metro is the stem meaning uterus. Endometritis, then, is a word which means inflammation __________ the uterus.

en"do-me-tri'tis

INTRA/ENDO

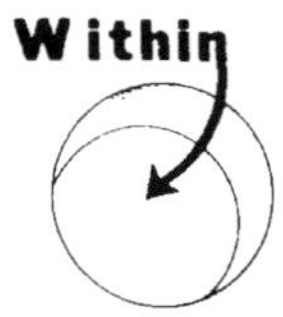

INTRA-ABDOMINAL
ENDOMETRITIS

inside/within

****

142 Peri- is a prefix which means around or surrounding. Cardio is the stem for heart. Pericarditis, then, is a word which means inflammation __________ the heart.

per"i-kar-di'tis

PERI

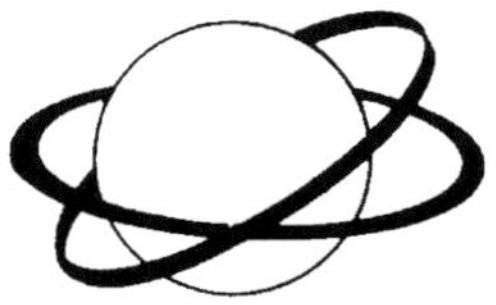

PERICARDITIS

around/surrounding

****

143 Ec- and ecto- are prefixes which mean out and outside. An ectopic pregnancy, for example, is a pregnancy which occurs __________ the uterine cavity.

ek-top'ik

EC/ECTO

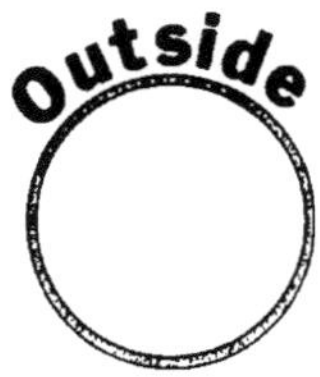

ECTOPIC PREGNANCY

outside

****

144 Em- and en- are also prefixes which mean within or inside. Empyema, for example, means pus __________ a body cavity.

em"pi-e'mah

EM/EN

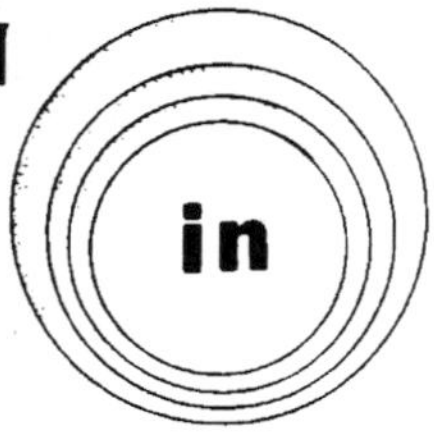

EMPYEMA

inside/within

****

145 Retro- and post- are prefixes which mean behind. Retrocardial means located __________ the heart and postnasal means situated __________ the nose.

ret"ro-kar'de-al
post-na'zal

RETRO/POST

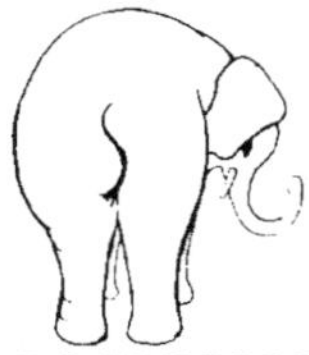

RETROCARDIAL
POSTNASAL

behind, behind

****

146 The prefixes sub- and hypo- mean under. Subcutaneous, for example, means __________ the skin, and a hypodermic needle is one that is inserted __________ the skin.

sub"ku-ta'ne-us
hi"po-der'mik

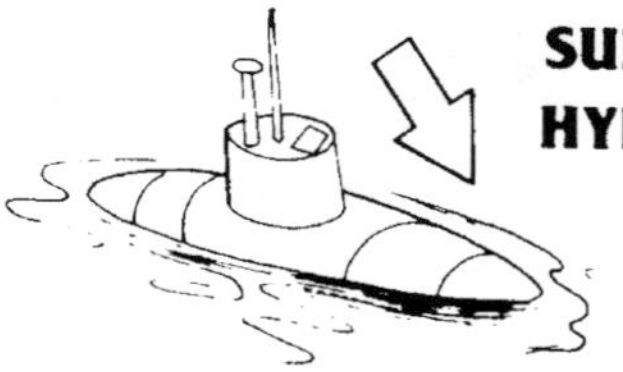

SUB / HYPO

SUBCUTANEOUS
HYPODERMIC

under, under

****

147 Inter- is a prefix meaning between. The stem, costal, means ribs. Therefore, intercostal muscles are muscles which are ___________ the ribs.

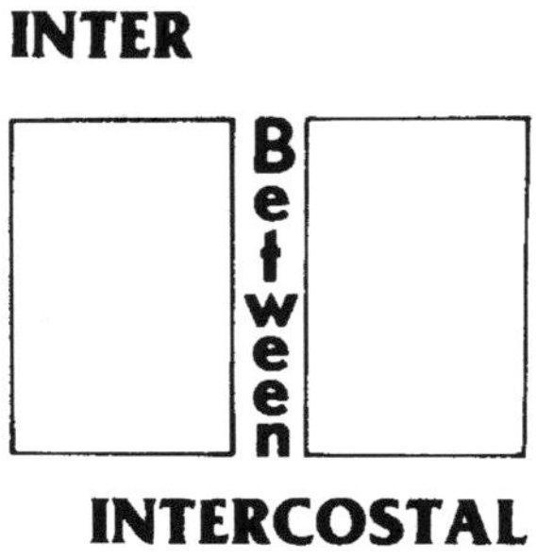

in"ter-kos'tal

between

****

148 In review, given the meaning of each of the following prefixes which indicate location:

a. intra-/endo-: ___________

inside/within (frames 140 & 141)

****

b. peri-: ___________

around/surrounding (frame 142)

****

c. ec-/ecto-: ___________

out/outside (frame 143)

****

d. em-/en-: ___________

within/inside (frame 144)

****

e. retro-/post-: ___________

behind (frame 145)

****

f. sub-/hypo-: ___________

under (frame 146)

****

g. inter-: ___________

between (frame 147)

****

149 To further reinforce what you have learned, write the correct word in each of the blanks in the following sentences:

a. The dash after intra- indicates that the stem comes __________ (before, after) the prefix.

after (frame 139)

****

b. Intra-abdominal means __________ the abdomen.

inside/within (frame 140)

****

c. Endometritis means inflammation __________ the uterus.

inside/within (frame 141)

****

d. Pericarditis means inflammation __________ the heart.

around (frame 142)

****

e. Ectopic pregnancy is one which occurs __________ the uterine cavity.

outside (frame 143)

****

f. Empyema is a condition where there is an accumulation of pus __________ a body cavity.

inside/within (frame 144)

****

g. Retrocardial means located __________ the heart.

behind (frame 145)

****

h. Postnasal means situated
__________ the nose.

behind (frame 145)

****

i. Subcutaneous indicates
__________ the skin.

under (frame 146)

****

j. A hypodermic needle is one that is
inserted __________ the skin.

under (frame 146)

****

k. Intercostal muscles are muscles
which are __________ the ribs.

between (frame 147)

****

> If you missed any of the questions in frames 148 and 149, please review the appropriate frame(s) before continuing to frame 150.

Section IV. PREFIXES - PERTAINING TO TIME

We will now study the prefixes that indicate time.

****

150 The prefixes ante- and pre- mean before. By combining the prefix ante- with the stem partum, you know that antepartum means __________ childbirth.

an'te-par'tum

ANTE/PRE

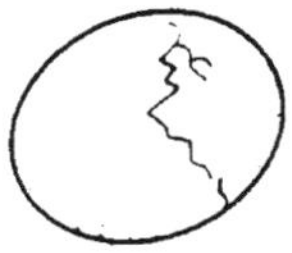

ANTEPARTUM
PREOPERATIVE

before

****

151 A <u>pre</u>operative medication is a medication which is given __________ (before, during, after) surgery.

pre-op'er-a-tiv

ANTE/PRE

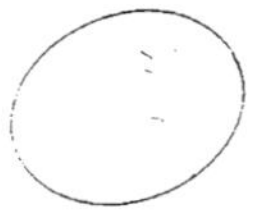

ANTEPARTUM
PREOPERATIVE

before

****

152 The prefix <u>post</u>- also means after. Consequently, a <u>post</u>operative complication is a complication which occurred (before, during, after) surgery.

post-op'er-a-tiv

POST

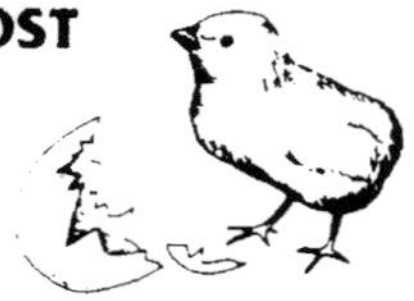

POST PARTUM
POSTOPERATIVE

after

****

153 In review, give the meaning of each of the following prefixes which indicate time:

a. ante-: __________

before (frame 150)

****

b. pre-: __________

before (frame 151)

****

c. post-: __________

after (frame 152)

****

154 To further reinforce what you have learned, please write the correct word in each of the blanks in the following sentences:

a. Antepartum means __________ childbirth.

before (frame 150)

****

b. A preoperative medication is one which is given __________ surgery.

before (frame 151)

****

c. A postoperative complication is one occurring __________ surgery.

after (frame 152)

****

> If you missed any of the questions in frames 153 and 154, please review the appropriate frame(s) before continuing to frame 155.

Section V: PREFIXES - PERTAINING TO NEGATION

We will now study prefixes that indicate negation.

****

155 The prefixes a- or- an mean without or absence of. Therefore, afebrile means __________ fever.

a-feb'ril

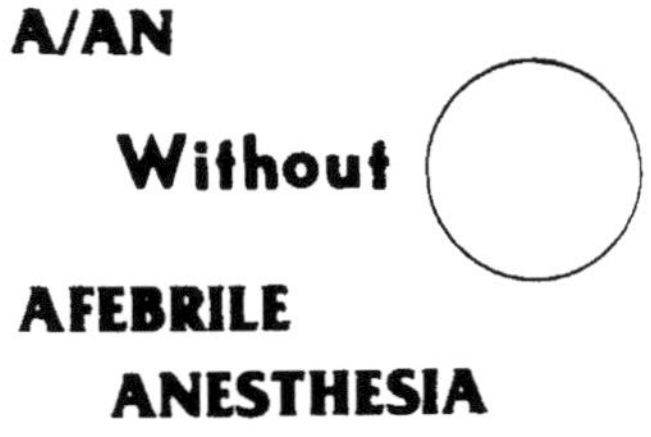

without/absence of

****

156 The stem esthesia means feeling. Therefore, anesthesia means __________ feeling.

an"es-the'ze-ah

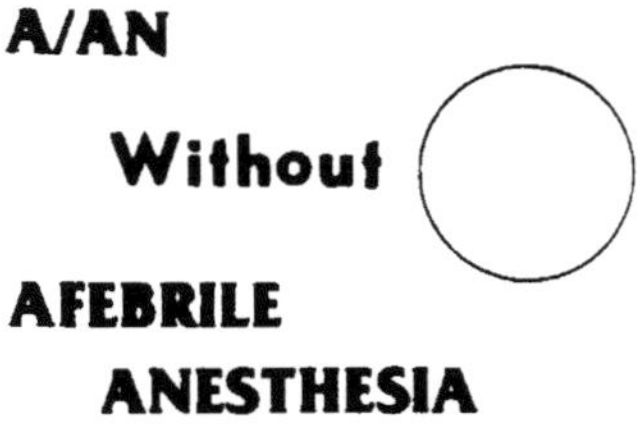

without

****

157 The prefix <u>anti</u>- means against. The term antitoxin means __________ toxin or poison.

an"ti-tok'sin

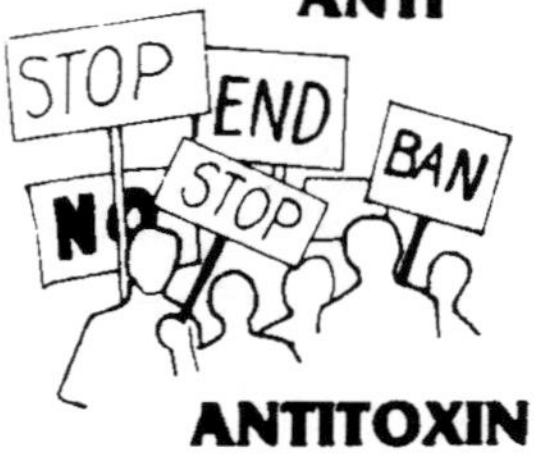

against

****

158 In review, give the meaning of each of the following prefixes which indicate negation:

a. a-: __________

without/absence of (frame 155)

****

b. an-: __________

without (frame 156)

****

c. anti-: __________

against (frame 157)

****

159 To further reinforce what you have learned, please write the correct word in each of the blanks in the following sentences:

a. Afebrile means __________ fever.

without/absence of (frame 155)

****

b. Anesthesia means __________ feeling.

without/absence of (frame 156)

****

c. Antitoxin means __________ toxin or poison.

against (frame 157)

****

If you missed any of the questions in frames 158 and 159, please review the appropriate frame(s) before continuing to frame 160.

Section VI. PREFIXES - PERTAINING TO AMOUNT OR COMPARISON

We will now study prefixes thatindicate amount or comparison.

****

160 Uni and mono- are prefixes which mean one or single. Monocyte, for example, refers to a __________ cell. A unicycle has one wheel.

mon'o-sit

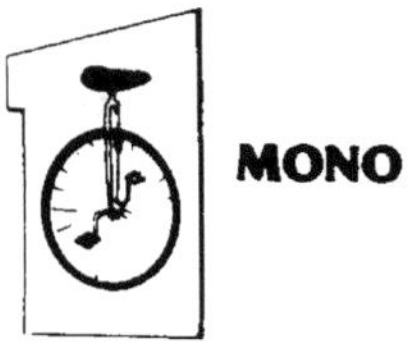

MONOCYTE

single

****

161 Bi- is a prefix indicating the number two. Bi-lateral, then, refers to __________ sides. A bicycle has two wheels.

bi-lat'er-al

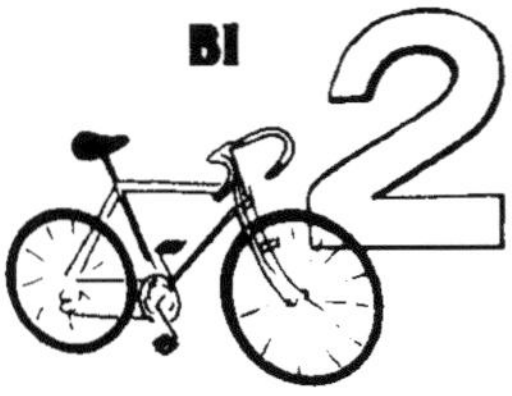

BILATERAL

two

****

162 The prefix for three is tri. Therefore, the valve in the heart which has __________ parts is called the tricuspid valve. A tricycle has three wheels.

tri-kus'pid

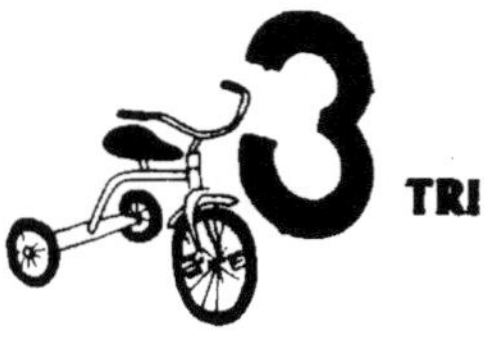

TRICUSPID

three

****

163 The prefix quadri- means four. A person with quadriplegia has paralysis in all __________ limbs.

kwod"ri-ple'je-ah

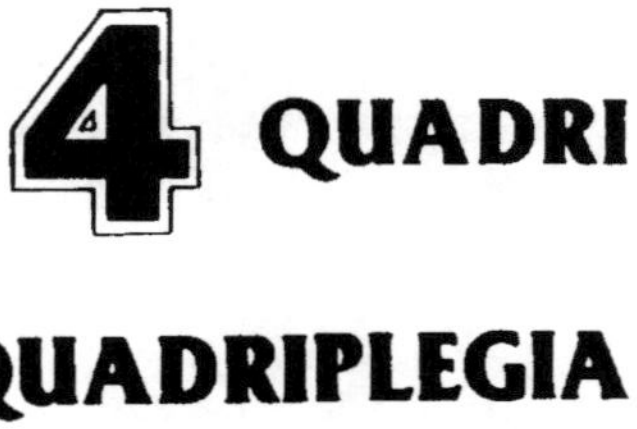

four

****

164 The prefixes multi- and poly- mean many or much. A person with polyneuritis has inflammation of __________ nerves.

pol"e-nu-ri'tis

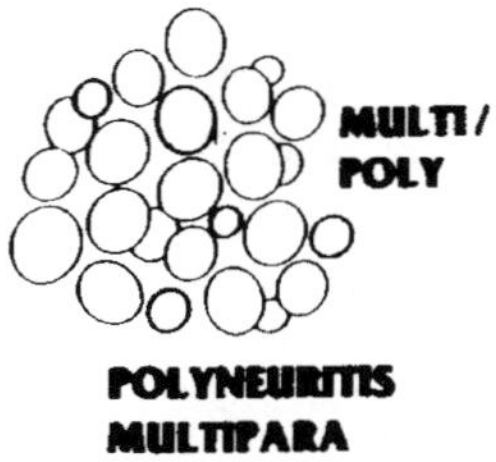

many

****

165 The prefixes hemi- and semi- mean half. A person with hemiplegia has paralysis on one-______ of the body.

hem"e-ple'je-ah

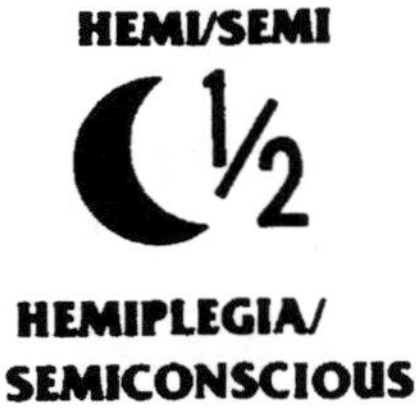

half

****

166 A person who is semiconscious is __________ conscious.

sem"e-kno'shus

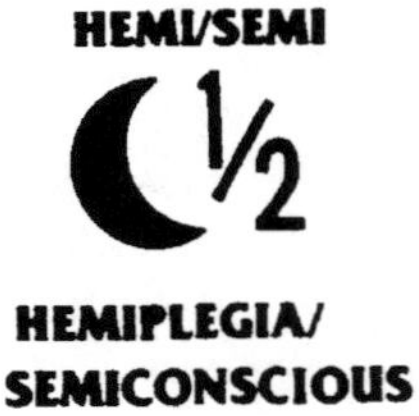

half

****

167 The prefix <u>hypo</u>- also means too little, or low. Therefore, a person with <u>hypo</u>tension has __________ blood pressure.

HYPO

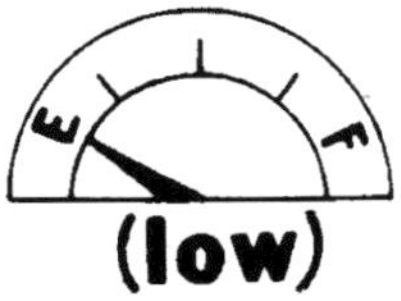

hi"po-ten'shun

HYPOTENSION

low

****

168 <u>Hyper</u>- is a prefix that is just the opposite of hypo-. Hyper means above or high. A person with <u>hyper</u>tension, then, has blood pressure above the normal or __________ blood pressure.

HYPER

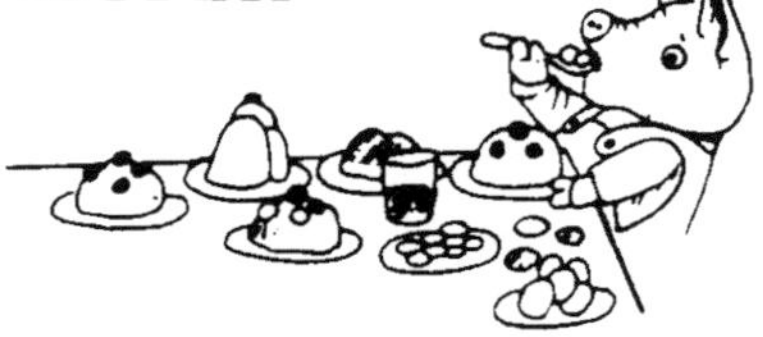

hi"per-ten'shun

HYPERTENSION

high

****

169 Emesis, as you know from lesson 2, is a word that means vomiting. A word that means excessive vomiting is __________ emesis.

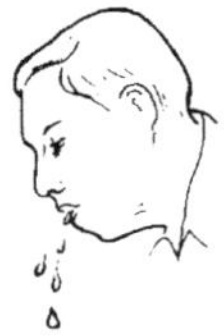

hi"per-em'e-sis

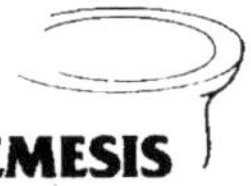

hyper

****

170 The prefix for fast is <u>tachy</u>-. A person with <u>tachy</u>cardia has an abnormally __________ heartbeat.

tak'e-kar'de-ah

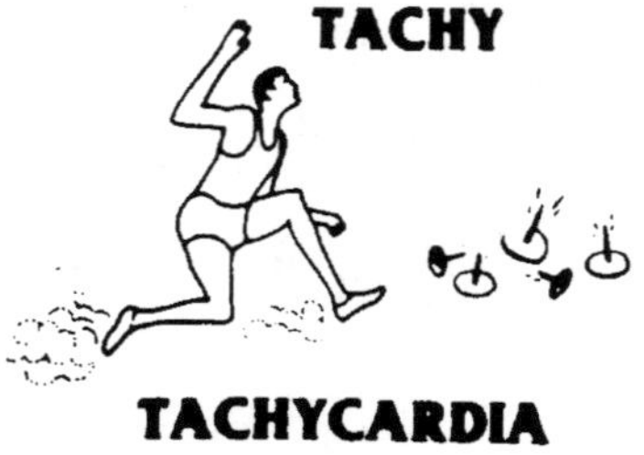

fast

****

171 The prefix for slow is <u>brady</u>-. A person with <u>brady</u>cardia has an abnormally __________ heartbeat.

brad"e-kar'de-ah

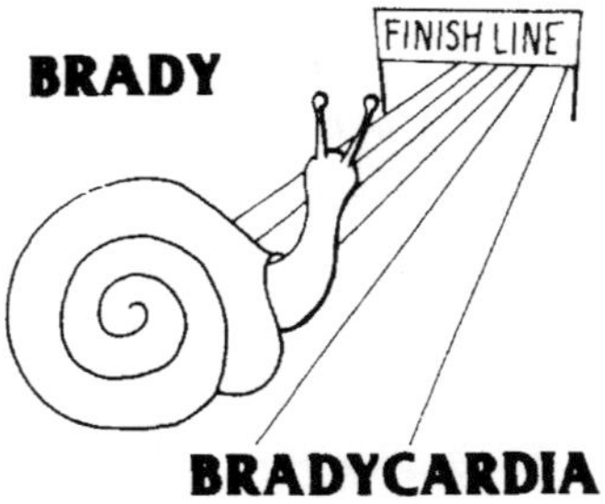

slow

****

172 The prefix for little or scanty is <u>oligo</u>-. The stem meaning urine is -uria. Therefore, <u>oliguria</u> means __________ or __________ urine.

ol"i-gu're-ah

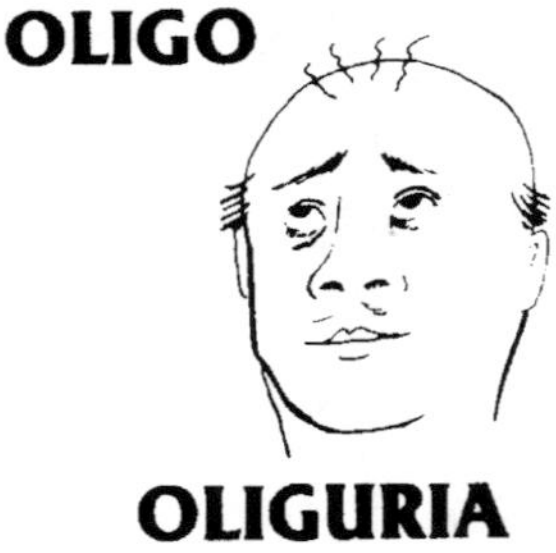

little/scanty

****

173 In review, give the meaning of each of the following prefixes which indicate amount or comparison:

a. Mono-: __________

one/single (frame 160)

****

b. Bi-: __________

two/double (frame 161)

****

c. Tri-: __________

three (frame 162)

****

d. Quadri: __________

four (frame 163)

****

e. Multi-/Poly-: __________

many/much (frame 164)

****

f. Hemi-/Semi-: __________

half (frame 165)

****

g. Hypo-: __________

low (frame 167)

****

h. Hyper-: __________

high (frame 168)

****

i. Tachy-: __________

fast (frame 170)

****

j. Brady-: __________

slow (frame 171)

****

k. Oligo-: __________

little/scanty (frame 172)

****

174 To further reinforce what you have learned, please write the correct word in each of the blanks in the following sentences.

a. Monocyte refers to a __________ cell.

single (frame 160)

****

b. Bilateral refers to ___________ sides.

two (frame 161)

****

c. The tricuspid valve in the heart has ___________ parts.

three (frame 162)

****

d. A person with quadriplegia has paralysis of ___________ limbs.

four (frame 163)

****

e. The medical term polyneuritis indicates inflammation of ___________ nerves.

many (frame 164)

****

f. When a person has hemiplegia, he has paralysis on one-___________ of the body.

half (frame 165)

****

g. A person who is semiconscious is ___________ conscious.

half (frame 165)

****

h. A person with hypotension has ___________ blood pressure.

low (frame 167)

****

i. A person with hypertension has
__________ blood pressure.

high (frame 168)

****

j. Tachycardia indicates an abnormally
__________ heartbeat.

fast (frame 170)

****

k. Bradycardia refers to an abnormally
__________ heartbeat.

slow (frame 171)

****

l. Oliguria means __________ urine.

little/scanty (frame 172)

****

If you missed any of the questions in frames 173 and 174, please review the appropriate frame(s) before continuing to frame 175.

Section VII. PREFIXES - PERTAINING TO COLOR

We will now study the prefixes that indicate color.

****

175 The prefix leuko- means white. A leukocyte, then, refers to a __________ blood cell.

lu'ko-sit

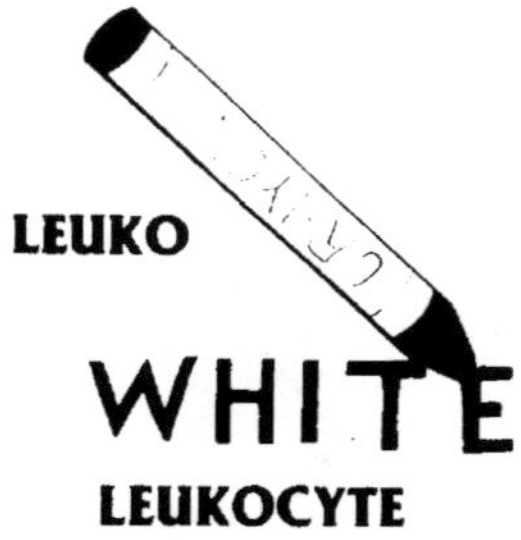

white

****

176 Erythro- is a prefix meaning red. An erythrocyte, therefore, refers to a __________ blood cell.

e-rith'ro-sit

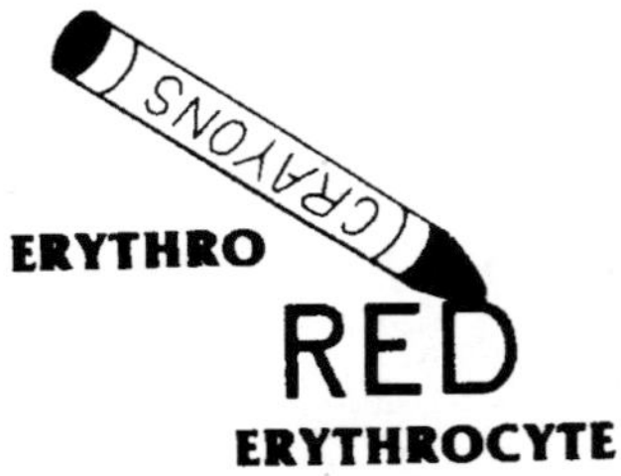

red

****

177 Cyano- is a prefix meaning blue. Cyanosis refers to a __________ condition of the skin.

si"ah-no'sis

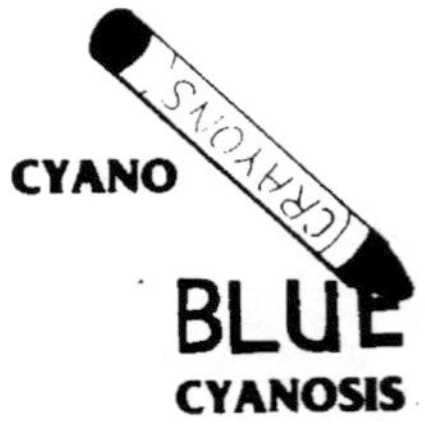

blue/bluish

****

178 Melano- is a prefix meaning dark or black. A melanoma is a malignant or __________ tumor.

MELANO

MELANOMA

mel"ah-no'mah

dark/black

****

An Invitation to Your Love

Oh! Beauty rare with eyes cyano,
Shimmering, shining hair melano,
Pearly teeth, and lips erythro,
Cheeks where only peaches will grow,
Warm and lovely skin so leuko,
Come with me into my nook-o?

179 In review, give the meaning of each of the following prefixes which indicates color.

a. Leuko-: __________

white (frame 175)

****

b. Erythro-: __________

red (frame 176)

****

c. Cyano-: __________

blue (frame 177)

****

d. Melano-: __________

dark/black (frame 178)

****

180 To further reinforce what you have learned, please write the correct word in each of the blanks in the following sentences.

a. A leukocyte is a __________ blood cell.

white (frame 175)

****

b. An erythrocyte is a __________ blood cell.

red (frame 176)

****

c. Cyanosis is a __________ condition of the skin.

blue (frame 177)

****

d. When someone has a melanoma, he has a malignant __________ mole or tumor.

dark/black (frame 178)

****

If you missed any of the questions in frames 179 and 180, please review the appropriate frame(s) before continuing to frame 181.

Section VIII. PREFIXES - PERTAINING TO SIZE AND POSITION

We will now study the prefixes thatindicate size.

****

181 Micro- is a prefix meaning small. A cyte is a stem meaning cell. A microcyte, therefore, is a very __________ cell.

mi'kro-sit

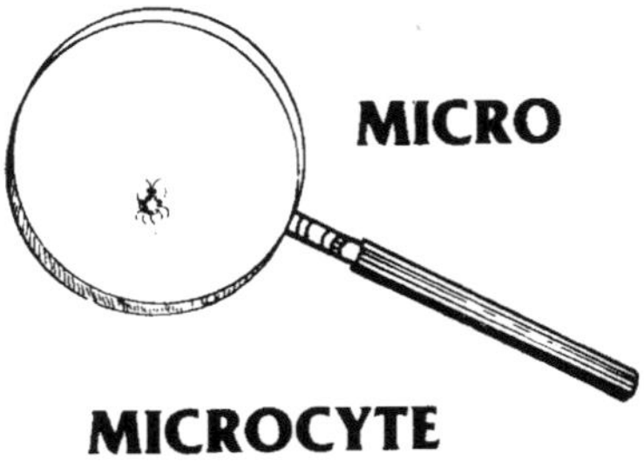

small

****

182 A word indicating smallness of heart is __________cardia.

mi"kro-kar'de-ah

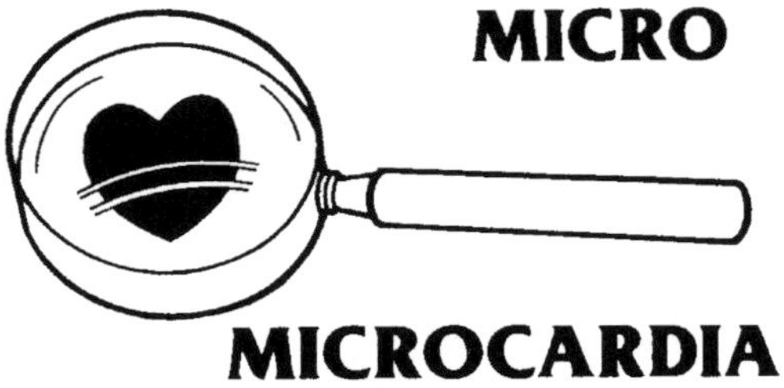

microcardia

****

183 Macro- is a prefix which means the opposite of micro. Macro- is used in words to mean __________.

mak'ro-sit

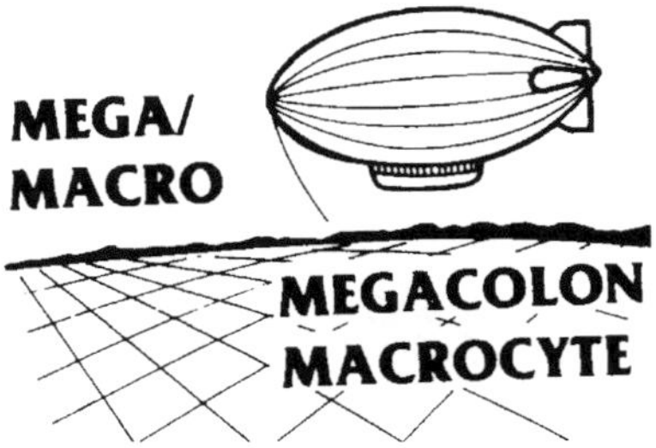

large

****

184 Things that are macroscopic can be seen with the naked eye. Very large cells are called __________cytes.

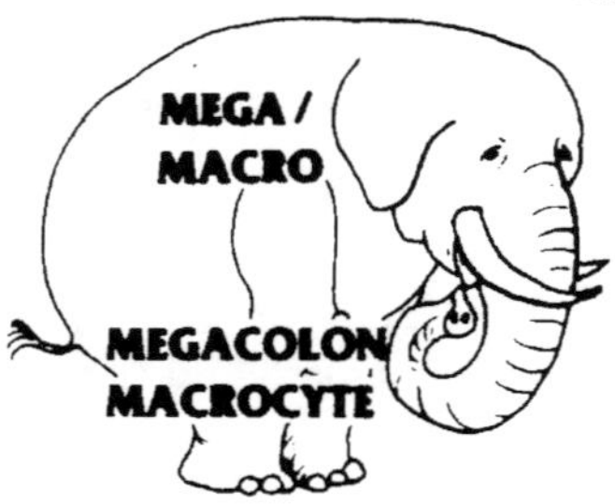

mak"ro-scop'ik

macrocytes

****

185 Mega- is also a prefix which means large. A megacolon is an abnormally __________ colon.

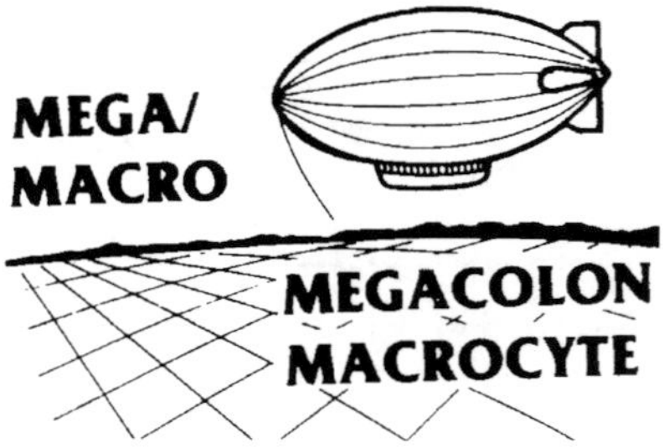

meg"ah-ko'lon

large

****

We will now study the prefixes that indicate position.

****

186 Antero- is a prefix meaning anterior part or in front of. Latero- is a prefix meaning side. Therefore, anterolateral means situated in __________ and to one _________.

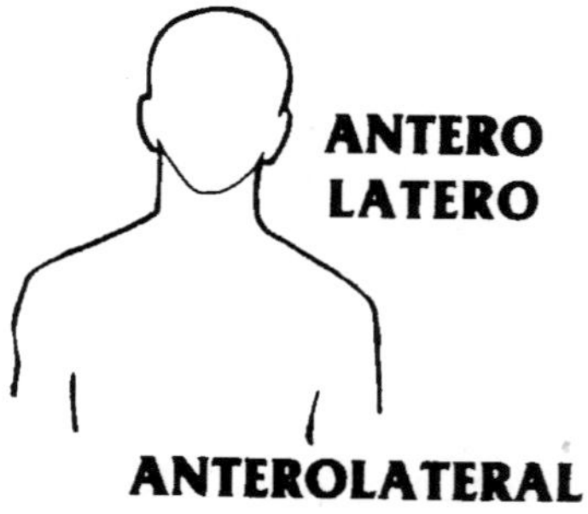

an"ter-o-lat'er-al

front/side

****

187 Dextro- is a prefix which means to the right. Dextrocardia, therefore, refers to having the heart on the __________ side of the body.

deks"tro-kar'de-ah

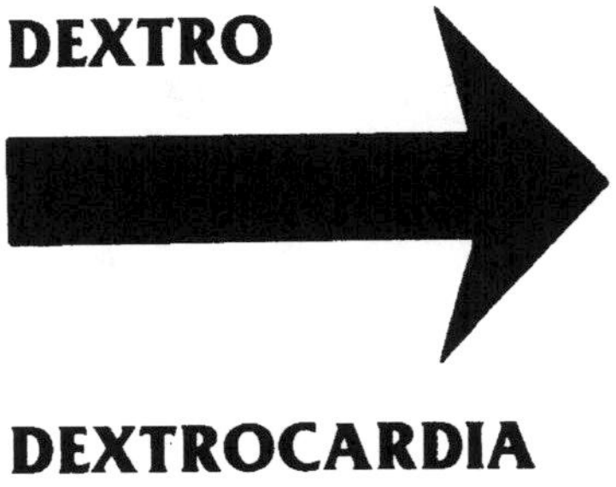

right

****

188 Levo- is a prefix meaning to the left. Levoversion is a term which means the act of turning to the __________.

le"vo-ver'zhun

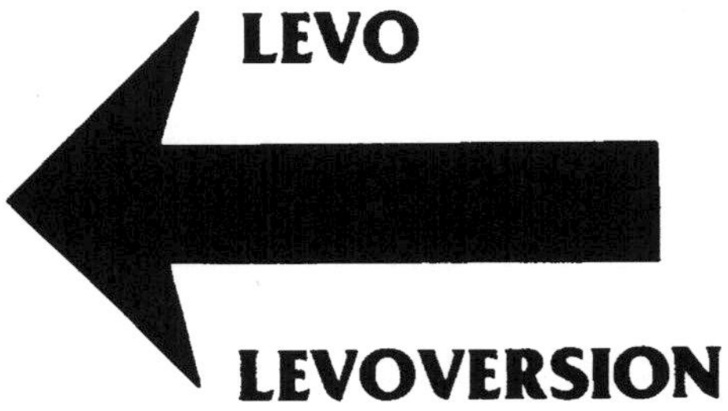

left

****

189 Medio- is a prefix meaning middle. The medial part of the body pertains to the __________.

me'de-al

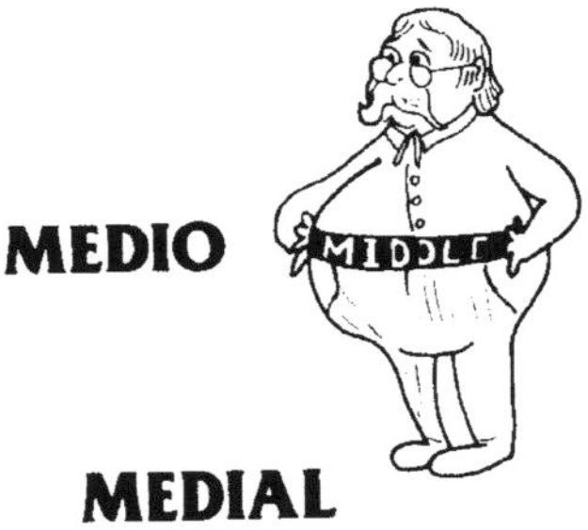

middle

****

190 In review, give the meaning of each of the following prefixes which indicate size and position.

a. Micro: __________

small (frame 181)

****

b. Macro-: __________

large (frame 183)

****
c. Mega-: __________

large (frame 185)

****
d. Antero-: __________

to the front (frame 186)

****
e. Latero-: __________

to the side (frame 186)

****
f. Dextro-: __________

to the right (frame 187)

****
g. Levo-: __________

to the left (frame 188)

****
h. Medio-: __________

middle (frame 189)

****
191 To further reinforce what you have learned, please write the correct word in each blank in the following sentences.

a. A microcyte is a very __________ cell.

small (frame 181)

****
b. Macrocytes are very __________ cells.

large (frame 183)

****

c. A person with a megacolon has an abnormally __________ colon.

large (frame 185)

****

d. Anterolateral means in __________ and to one __________.

front/side (frame 186)

****

e. If the heart is on the __________ side of the body, it is referred to as dextrocardia.

right (frame 187)

****

f. Levoversion means the act of turning to the __________.

left (frame 188)

****

g. The medial part of the body is called the __________ part.

middle (frame 189)

****

If you missed any of the questions in frames 190 and 191, please review the appropriate frame(s) before continuing to frame 192.

Section IX. PREFIXES - PERTAINING TO MISCELLANEOUS ITEMS

We will now conclude our study of the prefixes with some miscellaneous ones.

****

192 Hydro- is a prefix meaning water. Hydrophobia, then, means fear of __________.

hi"dro-fo'be-ah

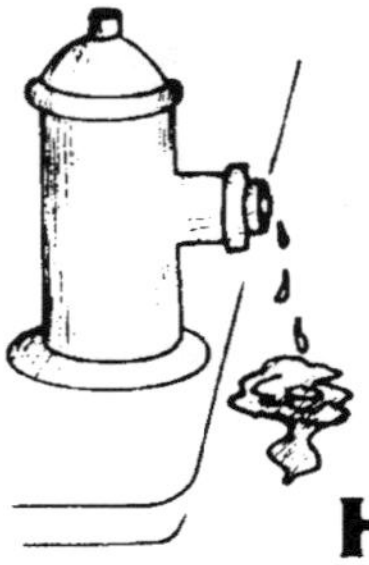

HYDRO

HYDROPHOBIA

water

****

193 Dys- is a prefix meaning difficult or painful. A patient with dyspnea would be experiencing __________ or __________ breathing.

disp'ne-ah

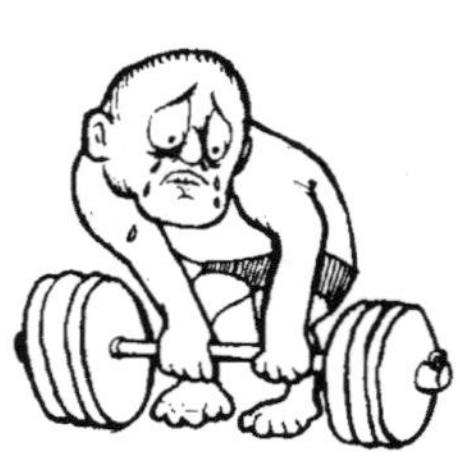

DYS

DYSPNEA

difficult/painful

****

194 Nox- and noct- are prefixes meaning night. Nocturia, therefore, means urination during the __________.

nok-tu're-ah

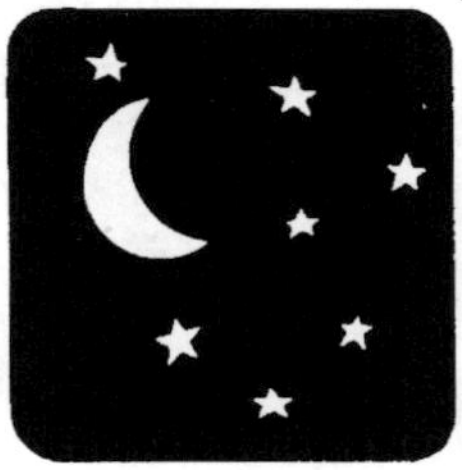

NOX / NOCT

NOCTURIA

night

****

195 Mal- is a prefix meaning bad. Malodorous means having a __________ odor.

mal-o'der-es

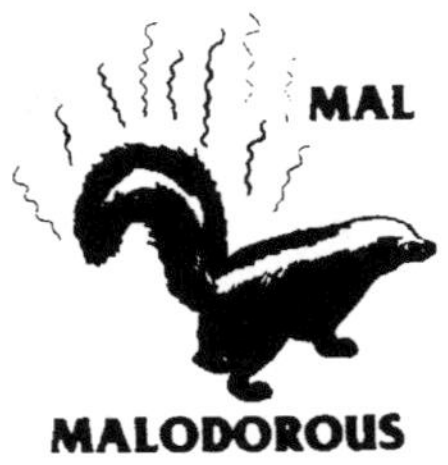

bad

****

196 Pan- is a prefix meaning total or all. A panhysterectomy, therefore, is a __________ hysterectomy.

pan"his-ter-ek'to-me

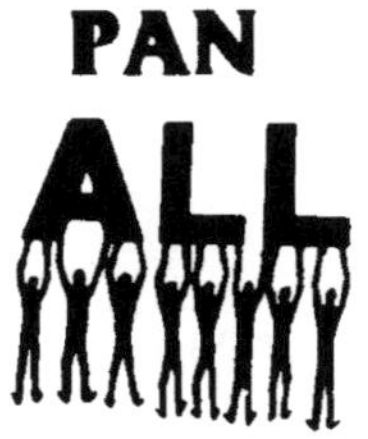

PANHYSTERECTOMY

total

****

197 In review, give the meaning of each of the following prefixes.

a. Hydro-: __________

water (frame 192)

****

b. Dys-: __________

difficult/painful (frame 193)

****

c. Nox/Noct-: __________

night (frame 194)

****

d. Mal-: __________

bad (frame 195)

****

e. Pan-: __________

all or total (frame 196)

****

198 To further reinforce what you have learned, please write the correct word in each blank in the following sentences.

a. A person with hydrophobia has a ___________ of water.

fear (frame 192)

****

b. A patient with dyspnea would be experiencing ___________ or ___________ breathing.

difficult/painful (frame 193)

****

c. Nocturia means urination at ___________.

night (frame 194)

****

d. If something is malodorous, it has a ___________ odor.

bad (frame 195)

****

e. A panhysterectomy is a ___________ hysterectomy.

total (frame 196)

****

If you missed any of the questions in frames 197 and 198, please review the appropriate frame(s) before continuing.

Continue with Self-Assessment

Section X. SELF-ASSESSMENT #2

You have now completed lesson 3. To evaluate how well you have learned the prefixes covered in lesson 3, complete the self-assessment #2 questions. This self-assessment is to assist you in determining whether you need to go back and review parts of lesson 3 before going to lesson 4.

When you have completed lesson 3 to your satisfaction, go to lesson 4.

SELF-ASSESSMENT #2

Prefixes

LISTED BELOW IN COLUMN "A" ARE 10 OF THE 50 LATIN AND GREEK PREFIXES GIVEN TO YOU. IN COLUMN "B" ARE THE ENGLISH MEANINGS OF THESE PREFIXES. MATCH THE TWO, AND WRITE THE ENGLISH MEANING FROM COLUMN "B" IN COLUMN "A."

EXAMPLE: BI = TWO

	COLUMN A			COLUMN B
1.	____________ HYPO		A.	BETWEEN
2.	____________ NOX, NOCT		B.	LOW/UNDER
3.	____________ POLY		C.	DIFFICULT/PAINFUL
4.	____________ CYANO		D.	FAST
5.	____________ INTER		E.	AROUND/SURROUNDING
6.	____________ PERI		F.	ONE
7.	____________ DYS		G.	EXCESSIVE/TOO MUCH
8.	____________ TACHY		H.	MANY/MUCH
9.	____________ MONO		I.	BLUE
10.	____________ HYPER		J.	NIGHT

SELF-ASSESSMENT QUIZ #2

PREFIXES

FOR EACH OF THE MULTIPLE CHOICE QUESTIONS BELOW, SELECT THE ONE MOST APPROPRIATE ANSWER. CIRCLE THE ANSWER.

11. THE PREFIX "SUB" IN THE WORD SUBCUTANEOUS MEANS:

    A. OVER
    B. RIB
    C. UNDER
    D. JOINT

12. THE PREFIX "BRADY" IN THE WORD BRADYCARDIA MEANS:

    A. FAST
    B. SLOW
    C. LOW
    D. FEW

13. THE PREFIX "HYDRO" IN THE WORD HYDROPHOBIA MEANS:

    A. AIR
    B. LIQUID
    C. GAS
    D. WATER

14. THE PREFIX "A" IN THE WORD AFEBRILE MEANS:

    A. WITHOUT
    B. WITHIN
    C. IN
    D. AROUND

15. THE PREFIX "TACHY" IN THE WORD TACHYCARDIA MEANS:

    A. LOW
    B. FAST
    C. SLOW
    D. FEW

16. THE PREFIX "ERYTHRO" IN THE WORD ERYTHROCYTE MEANS:

    A. BLUE
    B. WHITE
    C. RED
    D. BLACK

17. THE PREFIX "AN" IN THE WORD ANESTHESIA MEANS:

    A. WITHIN
    B. WITHOUT
    C. IN
    D. OUT

SELF-ASSESSMENT QUIZ #2

PREFIXES

18. THE PREFIX "OLIGO" IN THE WORD OLIGURIA MEANS:

    A. FEW/SCANTY
    B. LARGE
    C. SMALL
    D. MANY/MUCH

19. THE PREFIX "DEXTRO" IN THE WORD DEXTROCARDIA MEANS:

    A. RIGHT
    B. LEFT
    C. MIDDLE
    D. SIDE

20. THE PREFIX "EM" IN THE WORD EMPYEMA MEANS:

    A. BETWEEN
    B. UNDER
    C. OUT
    D. IN

Check your answers on the following pages

SOLUTIONS FOR SELF-ASSESSMENT #2

1. B (LOW/UNDER) HYPO
2. J (NIGHT) NOX, NOCT
3. H (MANY/MUCH) POLY
4. I (BLUE) CYANO
5. A (BETWEEN) INTER
6. E (AROUND/SURROUNDING) PERI
7. C (DIFFICULT/PAINFUL) DYS
8. D (FAST) TACHY
9. F (ONE) MONO
10. G (EXCESSIVE/TOO MUCH) HYPER

SOLUTIONS FOR SELF-ASSESSMENT QUIZ #2

11. THE PREFIX "SUB" IN THE WORD SUBCUTANEOUS MEANS:

C. UNDER

12. THE PREFIX "BRADY" IN THE WORD BRADYCARDIA MEANS:

B. SLOW

13. THE PREFIX "HYDRO" IN THE WORD HYDROPHOBIA MEANS:

D. WATER

14. THE PREFIX "A" IN THE WORD AFEBRILE MEANS:

A. WITHOUT

15. THE PREFIX "TACHY" IN THE WORD TACHYCARDIA MEANS:

B. FAST

16. THE PREFIX "ERYTHRO" IN THE WORD ERYTHROCYTE MEANS:

C. RED

17. THE PREFIX "AN" IN THE WORD ANESTHESIA MEANS:

B. WITHOUT

18. THE PREFIX "OLIGO" IN THE WORD OLIGURIA MEANS:

A. FEW/SCANTY

19. THE PREFIX "DEXTRO" IN THE WORD DEXTROCARDIA MEANS:

A. RIGHT

20. THE PREFIX "EM" IN THE WORD EMPYEMA MEANS:

D. IN

SOLUTIONS TO PRETEST #2

1. Poor/bad
2. Night
3. Painful/difficult
4. Water
5. Large
6. Small
7. Black
8. Blue
9. Red
10. White
11. Scant
12. Slow
13. Fast or rapid
14. One
15. Free from/without
16. Excessive
17. Half
18. Many
19. Outside
20. Around
21. Under
22. Below
23. After
24. Outside
25. Against
26. Inside
27. Behind
28. Before
29. Before
30. Between
31. Two/both

Go to Lesson 4

Continue with Lesson 3

LESSON ASSIGNMENT

LESSON 4 Suffixes Pertaining to Medical Terminology.

LESSON ASSIGNMENT Lesson 4, frame numbers 199-245.

LESSON OBJECTIVES After completing this lesson, you should be able to:

Give 10 of the 35 Latin and Greek medical suffixes and a list of English meanings of these suffixes, write the English meaning in the space provided without error.

LESSON 4

Section I. PRETEST #3

Before you turn to frame 199 and begin work on your study of suffixes in medical terminology, complete pretest #3. The pretest contains 28 questions relating to medical terminology suffixes.

If you correctly answer 90% or more of the questions, you pass the pretest and should proceed to the final examination. A score of 90% on this pretest is 27 correct answers.

****

If you pass the pretest for lesson 2, lesson 3, and lesson 4, with 90% accuracy, go to the final examination

****

Write your answers in the space provided in each question.

1. Arthropathy is a ________________ of the joints.

2. Enterorrhagia means ___________ of the small intestine.

3. Angiosclerosis is the _____________ of blood vessels.

4. Osteomalacia means __________________ of the bone.

5. Lipolysis is the ______________________ of fat.

6. Gastrectasia is the ________________ of the stomach.

7. Cephalalgia is term for _______________ in the head.

8. Cyanemia means blue ________________________.

9. Myelocele is the protrusion or _______ of the spinal cord.

10. Dermatosis means any skin _____________________.

11. Oophoroma is an ovarian ______________________.

12. Encephalitis is ___________________ of the brain.

13. A cardiocentesis is a ________________ of the heart.

14. Rhinorrhea is a ________________ from the nose.

15. Pyeloplasty is the ______ ______ of the renal pelvis.

16. Spermapenia means a ______________ of spermatozoa.

17. A nephropexy is the _______________ of a kidney.

18. An arthrotomy is an _______________ into a joint.

19. Esophagoduodenostomy is a new ___________ between the esophagus and the duodenum.

20. A stomatoscopy is an ___________ of the mouth with an instrument.

21. Neurorrhaphy means _________________ a nerve.

22. Hysteroptosis is the ______________ of the uterus.

23. Hematophobia is an abnormal _____________ of blood.

24. Acromegaly means that the extremities are ___________.

25. Keratectasia means _______________ of the cornea.

26. Hypertrophy means ______________________.

27. Appendectomy is the surgical _________ of the appendix.

28. Hepatorrhexis is the ______________ of the liver.

Check your answers on page 4-32

Section II. SUFFIXES - GENERAL INFORMATION AND DISEASES

Suffixes are the final element which we will study in analyzing medical terms. Normally, when reading or breaking down a medical word, begin with the suffix.

****

199 When reading or breaking down a medical term, we usually begin with the __________.

suffix

****

200 A suffix is a letter or syllable at the end of a word which adds meaning to the word.

A letter or syllable at the end of a word which adds to its meaning is called a __________.

suffix

****

Like prefixes, suffixes could be placed into different categories of meaning.

201 Suffixes differ from prefixes, however, in that a suffix comes (before, after) the stem.

after

****

Most suffixes are in common use in English, but a few are peculiar to medicine. The suffixes most commonly used to indicate disease are -<u>itis</u>, meaning inflammation; -<u>oma</u>, meaning tumor; and -<u>osis</u>, meaning condition, usually morbid.

202 Suffixes commonly used to indicate disease are __________, __________, and __________.

itis/oma/osis

****

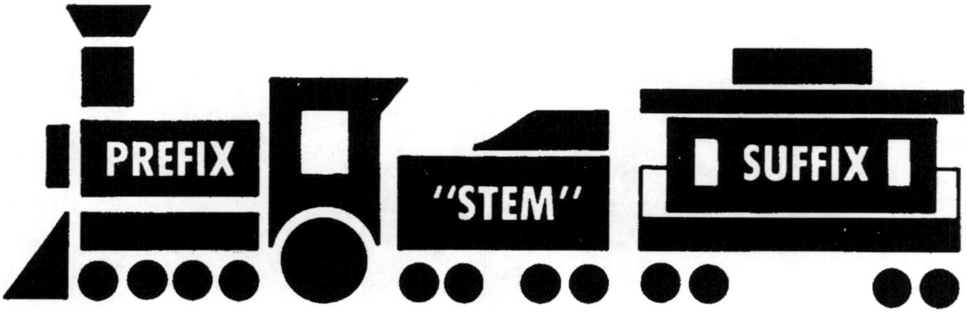

203 To further reinforce what you have learned, please write the correct word in each of the blanks in the following sentences:

a. A letter or syllable at the end of a word which adds to its meaning is called a __________.

suffix (frame 199)

****

b. When reading or breaking down a medical term, we usually begin with the __________.

suffix (frame 200)

****

c. Suffixes differ from prefixes in that a suffix comes __________ (before, after) the stem.

after (frame 201)

****

d. Suffixes commonly used to indicate disease are __________, __________, and __________.

itis/oma/osis (frame 202)

****

If you missed any of the questions in frame 203, please review the appropriate frame(s) before continuing to frame 204.

Section III. SUFFIXES - PERTAINING TO DIAGNOSIS

We will now look at the diagnostic suffixes.

****

204 The suffix -cele means hernia, protrusion, or tumor. A gastrocele, then, is a protrusion or __________ of the stomach.

gas'tro-sel

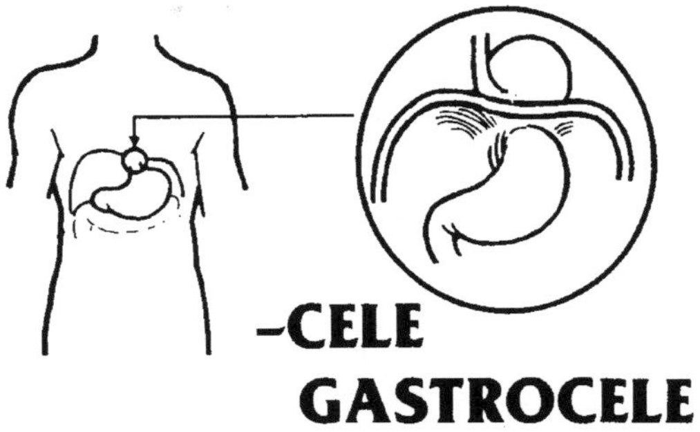

hernia

****

205 -Emia is the suffix for blood. A word we are all familiar with is leukemia, which is an abnormal amount of immature white blood cells. Hypoglycemia is a low amount of sugar in the __________.

lu-ke'me-ah
hi"po-gli-se'me-ah

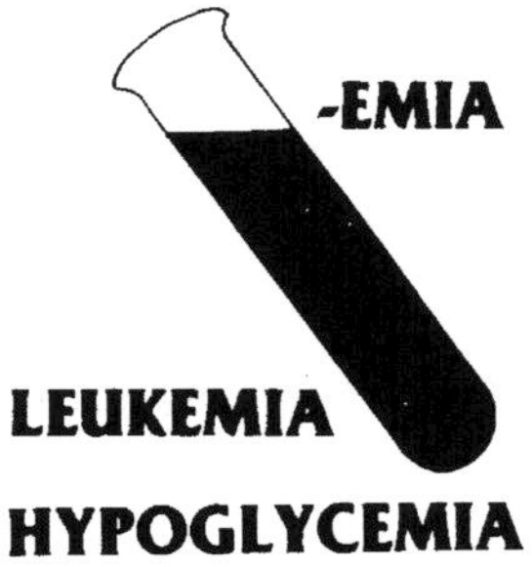

blood

****

206 -Ectasis and -ectasia are suffixes meaning dilation, dilatation, or expansion. Angiectasis, then, is abnormal __________ of a blood vessel.

an"je-ek'tah-sis

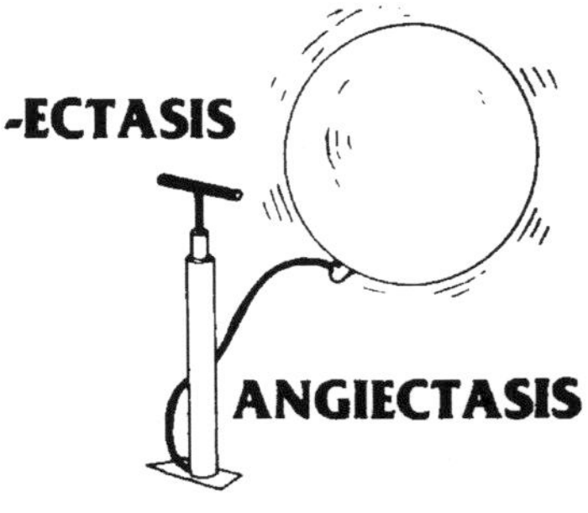

expanding/dilation/dilatation

****

207 The suffix for condition, formation of, or presence of is -iasis. Nephrolithiasis, therefore, is a __________ of stones in the kidney.

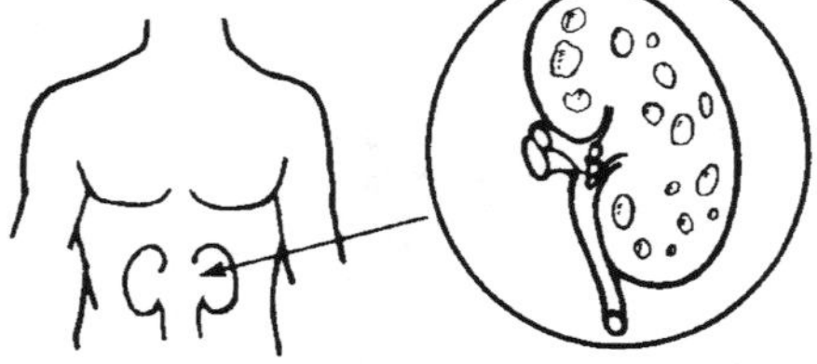

nef"ro-li-thi'ah-sis

condition

****

208 The suffix for inflammation is -itis. Encephalitis, then, is __________ of the brain.

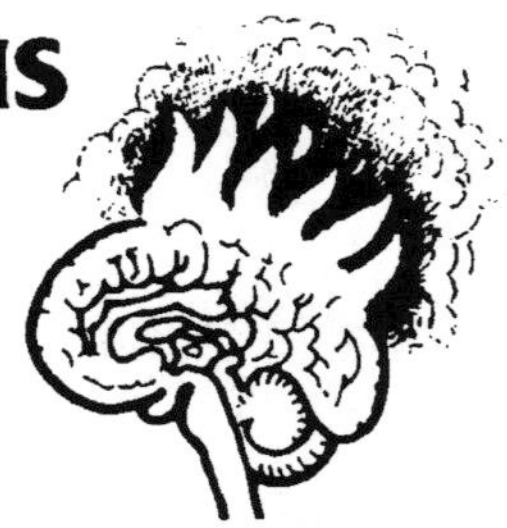

en"sef-ah-li'tis

inflammation

****

209 The suffix for softening is -malacia. Therefore, chondromalacia is __________ of the cartilage.

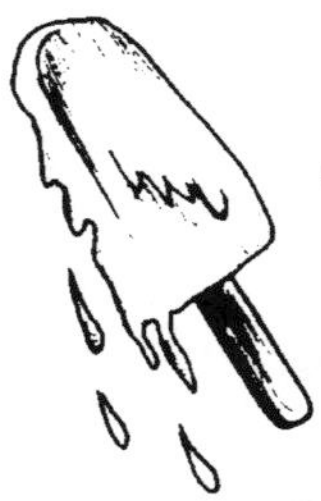

kon"dro-mah-la'she-ah

softening

****

210 The suffix for enlargement is -megaly. The stems for liver and spleen, as you will recall, are hepato and spleno. Hepatosplenomegaly, then, is __________ of the liver and spleen.

hep"ah-to-sple"no-meg'ah-le

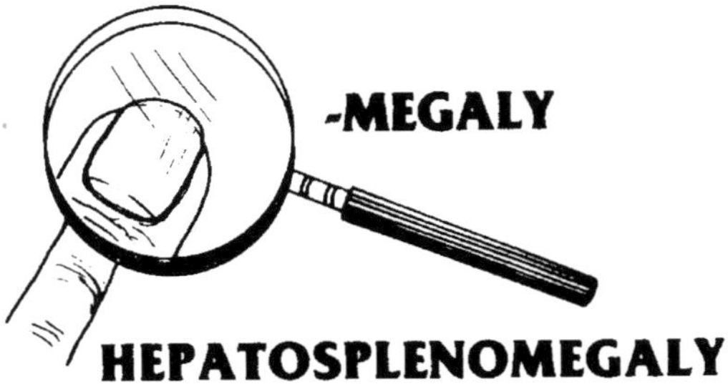

enlargement

****

211 The suffix for hardening is -sclerosis. The stem for artery, as you will recall, is arterio. Arteriosclerosis, then, is __________ of the arteries.

ar-te"re-o-skle-ro'sis

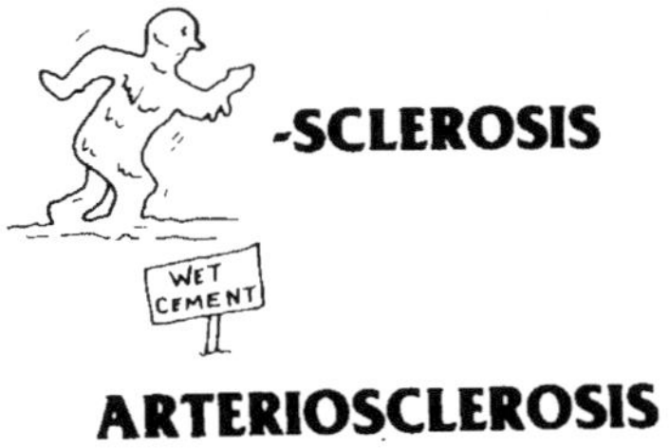

hardening

****

212 The suffix for tumor is -oma; thus a lipoma is a fatty __________.

li-po'mah

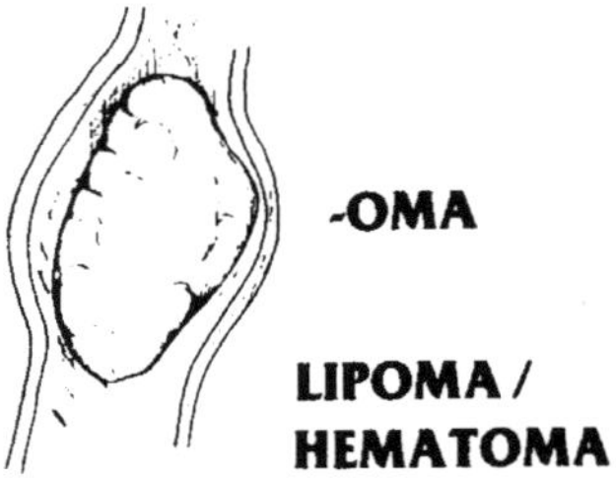

tumor

****

213 The suffix for condition or disease is -osis. Dermatophytosis, then, is a __________ of fungus of the skin.

der"mah-to-fi-to'sis

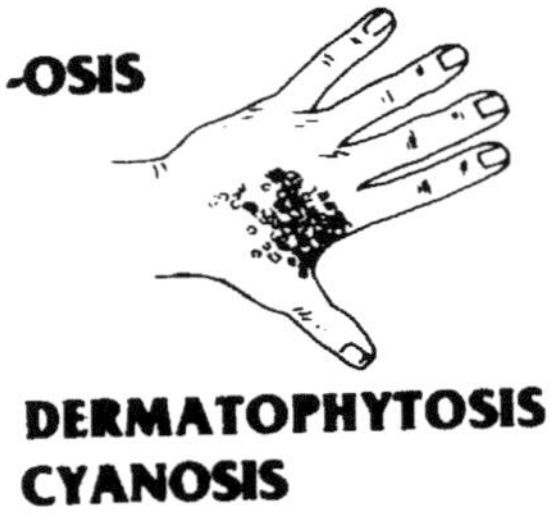

condition

****

214 The suffix for disease is -pathy. Thus, neuropathy is a __________ of the nerves.

nu-rop'ah-the

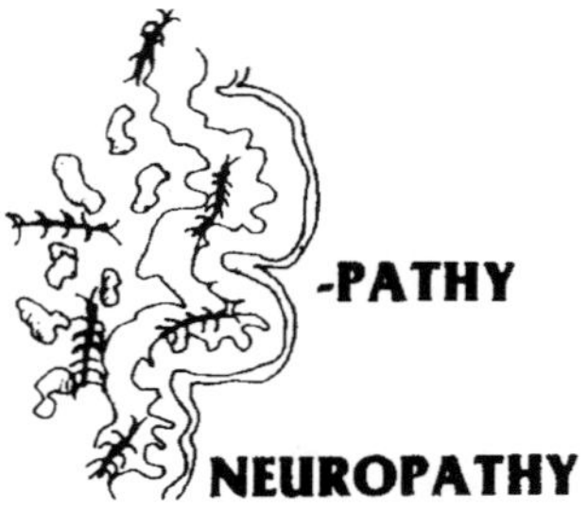

disease

****

215 The suffix for prolapse or downward displacement is ptosis. The stem for eyelid, as you will recall, is blepharo. Therefore, a blepharoptosis is a __________ __________ of the eyelid.

blef"ah-ro-to'sis

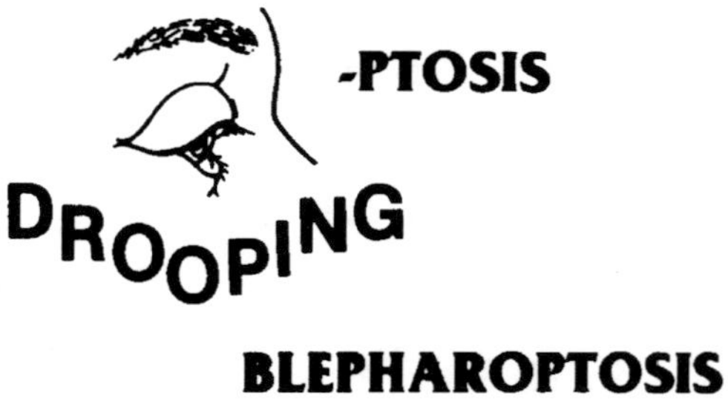

downward displacement

****

216 The suffix for rupture is -rrhexis. Cardiiiorrhexis, then, is a __________ of the heart.

kar"de-o-rek'sis

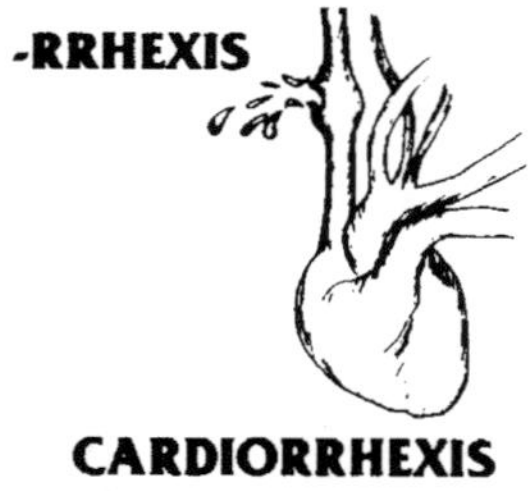

rupture

****

217 The suffix for growth or nourishment is -trophy. The medical term for excessive __________, then, is hypertrophy.

hi-per'tro-fe

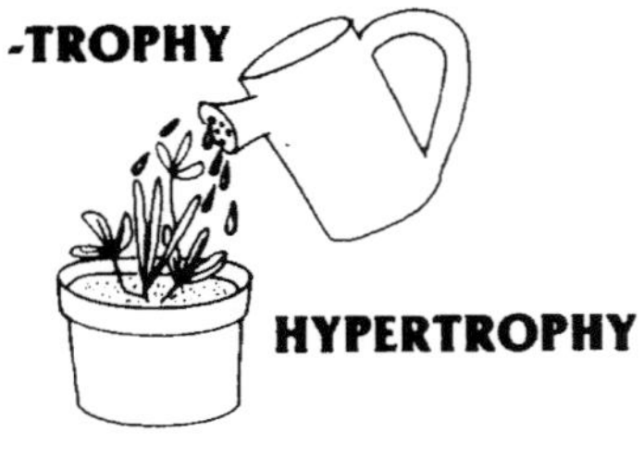

growth

****

218 The suffix for fear is -phobia. Hydrophobia, then, is a __________ of water.

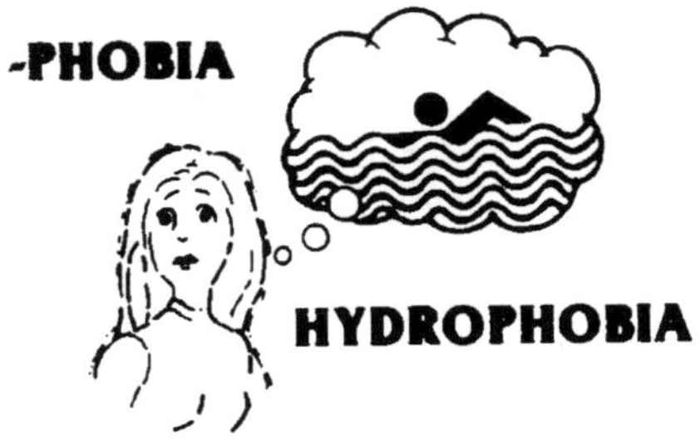

hi"dro-fo'be-ah

fear

****

219 In review, give the meaning of each of the following diagnostic suffixes:

a. -cele means: __________

hernia, protrusion, tumor (frame 204)

****

b. -emia means: __________

in the blood (frame 205)

****

c. -ectasis means: __________

dilation, dilatation, or expansion (frame 206)

****

d. -iasis means: __________

condition, formation of, presence of (frame 207)

****

e. -itis means: __________

inflammation (frame 208)

****

f. -malacia means: __________

softening (frame 209)

****

g. -megaly means: __________

enlargement (frame 210)

****

h. -sclerosis means: __________

hardening (frame 211)

****
i. -oma means: __________

tumor (frame 212)

****
j. -osis means: __________

condition (frame 213)

****
k. -pathy means: __________

disease (frame 214)

****
l. -ptosis means: __________

prolapse/downward displacement (frame 215)

****
m. -rrhexis means: __________

rupture (frame 216)

****
n. -trophy means: __________

growth/nourishment (frame 217)

****
o. -phobia means: __________

fear (frame 218)

****

220 To further review what you have learned, please write the correct word in each of the blanks in the following sentences.

a. A gastrocele is a protrusion or __________ of the stomach.

hernia (frame 204)

****

b. Hypoglycemia is a low amount of sugar in the __________.

blood (frame 205)

****

c. Angiectasis is abnormal __________ of a blood vessel.

dilation (frame 206)

****

d. Nephrolithiasis is a __________ of stones in the kidney.

dilation (frame 206)

****

e. Encephalitis is __________ of the brain.

inflammation (frame 208)

****

f. Chondromalacia is __________ of the cartilage.

softening (frame 209)

****

g. Hepatosplenomegaly is the __________ of the liver and spleen.

enlargement (frame 210)

****

h. Arteriosclerosis is __________ of the arteries.

hardening (frame 211)

****

i. A lipoma is a fatty __________.

tumor (frame 212)

****

j. Dermatophytosis is a fungus __________ of the skin.

condition (frame 213)

****

k. Neuropathy is a __________ of the nerves.

disease (frame 214)

****

l. Blepharoptosis is a __________ __________ of the eyelid.

downward displacement (frame 215)

****

m. Cardiorrhexis is a __________ of the heart.

rupture (frame 216)

****

n. Hypertrophy is the medical term for excessive __________.

growth (frame 217)

****

o. Hydrophobia is a __________ of water.

fear (frame 218)

****

If you missed any of the questions in frames 219 and 220, please review the appropriate frame(s) before continuing to frame 221.

Section IV. SUFFIXES - PERTAINING TO OPERATIVE PROCEDURES

Now let's look at the operative suffixes.

****

221 The suffix for removal or excision is -<u>ectomy</u>. The stem, salpingo, means tube, and the stem, oophoro, means ovary. A salpingo-oophor<u>ectomy</u>, therefore, is the __________ or __________ of tubes and ovaries.

sal-ping"go-o"of-o-rek'to-me

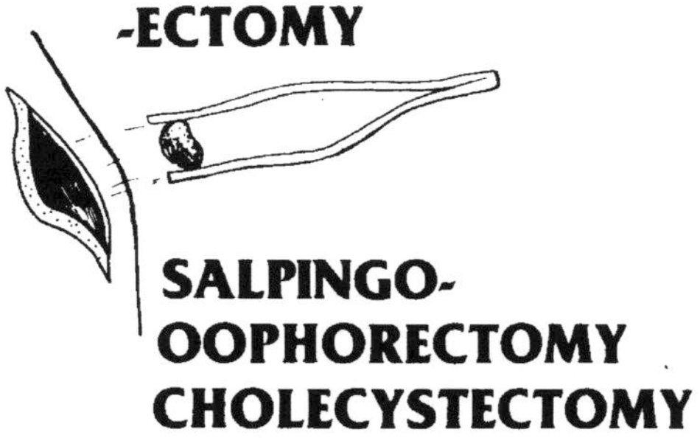

removal/excision

****

222 The stem cholecysto, as you recall, means gallbladder. Removal or excision of the gallbladder, therefore, is called a __________.

ko"le-sis-tek'to-me

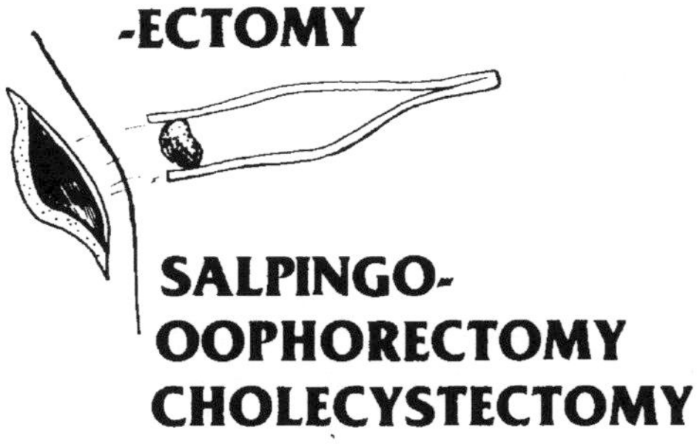

cholecystectomy

****

223 The suffix for inspection or examination is -<u>scopy</u>. A broncho<u>scopy</u>, then is an __________ of the bronchi.

brong-kos'ko-pe

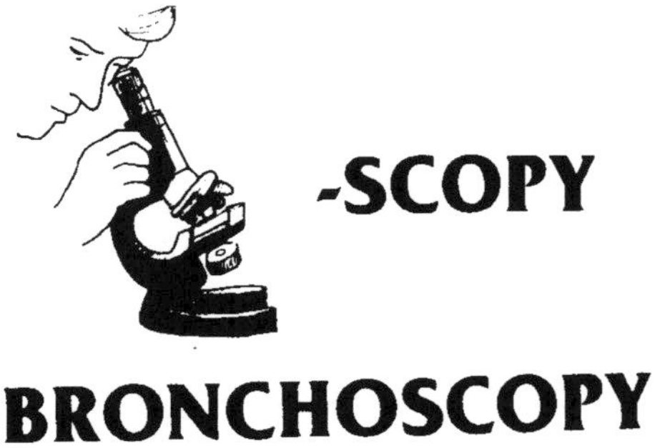

inspection/examination

****

224 -stomy is the suffix meaning surgical creation of an artificial opening. Therefore, a colostomy is an __________ into the colon.

ko-los'to-me

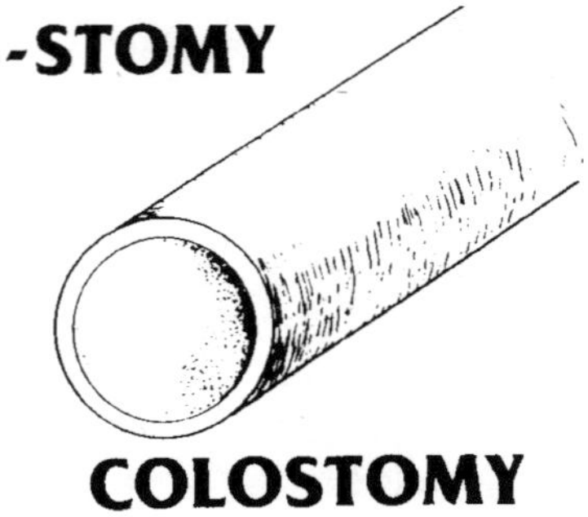

artificial opening

****

225 -tomy is the suffix meaning incision or cutting into. A laparotomy, then, is an __________ in the abdominal wall.

lap-ah-rot'o-me

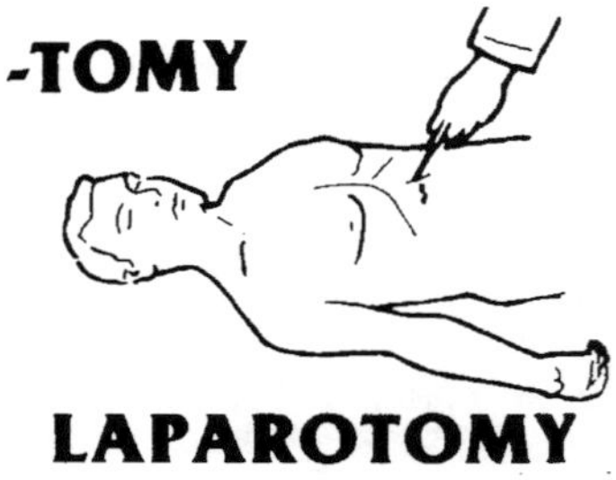

incision

****

226 The suffix for binding or fixation is -desis. Arthrodesis, then, is the medical term for surgical __________/__________ of a joint.

ar"thro-de'sis

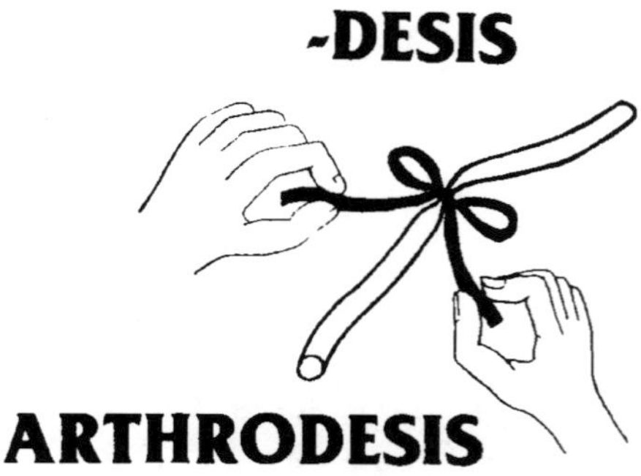

binding/fixation

****

227 The suffix for suspension or fixation is -pexy. An orchiopexy is __________ of an undescended testis.

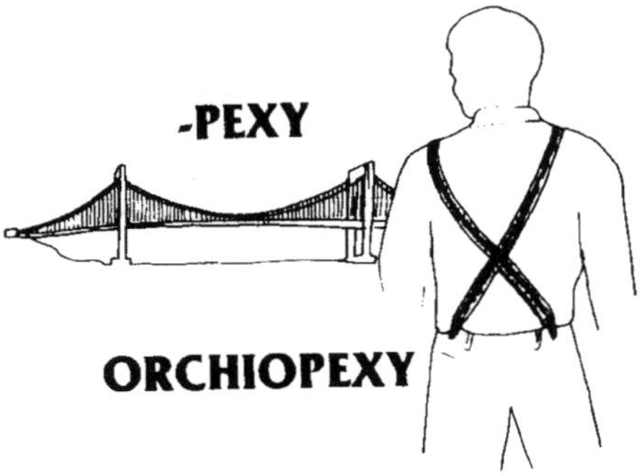

or"ke-o-pek'se

suspension/fixation

****

228 The suffix for plastic repair of is -plasty. Tympano, as you recall, is the stem for eardrum. Tympanoplasty, then, is the term for __________ __________ of the eardrum.

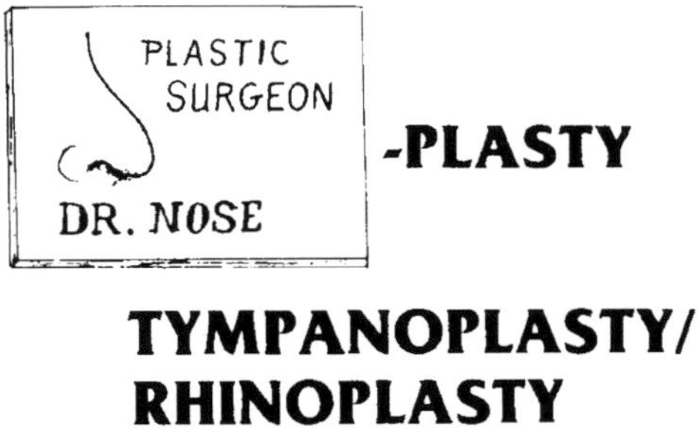

tim"pah-no-plas'te

plastic repair

****

229 The suffix -centesis means puncture. Arthrocentesis, therefore, means __________ of a joint for the removal of fluid.

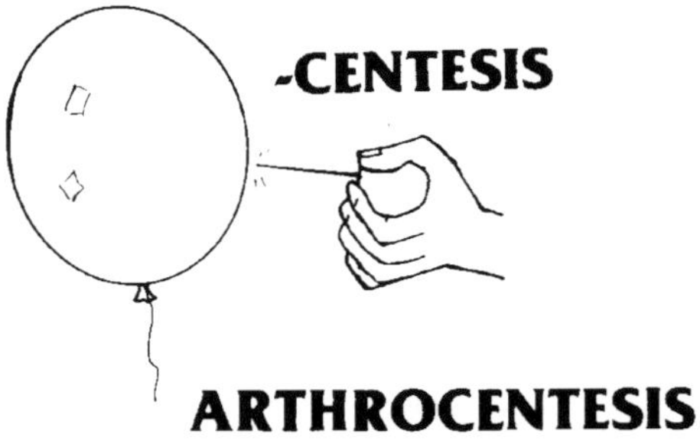

ar"thro-sen-te'sis

puncture

****

230 The suffix for suture repair is -rrhaphy. Neurorraphy is the medical term for __________ __________ of the nerve.

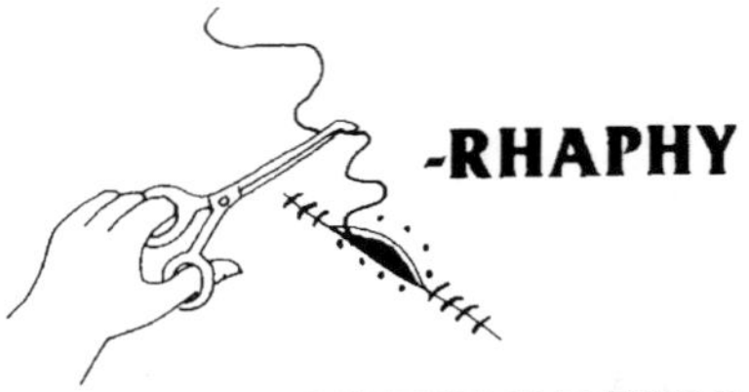

nu-ror'ah-fe

NEURORRHAPHY

suture repair

****

231 In review, write the meaning of each of the following operative suffixes in the blank provided.

a. -ectomy means: __________

removal/excision (frame 221)

****

b. -scopy means: __________

inspection/examination (frame 223)

****

c. -stomy means: __________

artificial opening into (frame 224)

****

d. -tomy means: __________

incision/cutting (frame 225)

****

e. -desis means: __________

binding/fixation (frame 226)

****

f. -pexy means: __________

suspension/fixation (frame 227)

****

g. -plasty means: __________

plastic repair (frame 228)

****

h. -centesis means: __________

puncture (frame 229)

****

i. -rrhaphy means: __________

suture repair (frame 230)

****

232 To further review what you have learned, please write the correct word in each of the blanks in the following sentences.

a. A salpingo-oophorectomy is the __________ or __________ of tubes and ovaries.

removal/excision (frame 221)

****

b. A bronchoscopy is an __________ of the bronchi.

examination/inspection (frame 223)

****

c. A colostomy is an __________ __________ __________ the colon.

artificial opening into (frame 224)

****

d. A laparotomy is an __________ into the abdominal wall.

incision (frame 225)

****

e. Arthrodesis is the medical term for a surgical __________ of a joint.

fixation (frame 226)

****

f. An orchiopexy is __________ of an undescended testis.

suspension/fixation (frame 227)

****

g. Rhinoplasty is the term for __________ __________ of the nose.

plastic repair (frame 228)

****

h. Arthrocentesis is removal of fluid from a joint by __________.

puncture (frame 229)

****

i. Neurorrhaphy is the __________ __________ of the nerve.

suture repair (frame 230)

****

If you missed any of the questions in frames 231 and 232, please review the appropriate frame(s) before continuing to frame 233.

Section V. SUFFIXES - PERTAINING TO SYMPTOMS

We will now study the symptomatic suffixes.

****

233 -algia is a suffix meaning pain. Dentalgia, then, is the medical term for a __________ in the tooth.

den-tal'je-ah

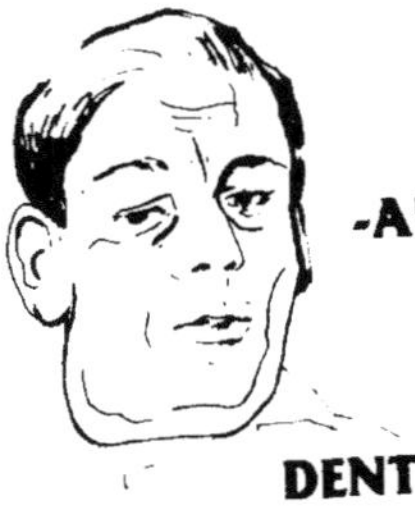

pain

****

234 -genic is the suffix for producing or originating. Pyo, as you recall, is the stem for pus. Pyogenic, then, is the term for __________ pus.

pi"o-jen'ik

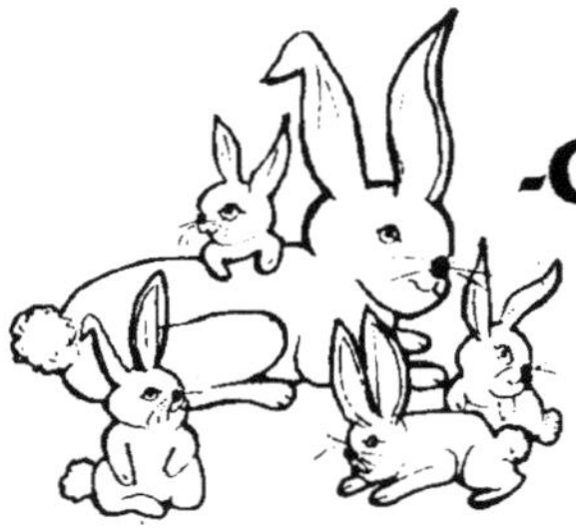

producing

****

235 -lysis is a suffix meaning destruction or breakdown. Hemolysis, therefore, means the __________ of red blood cells.

he-mol'i-sis

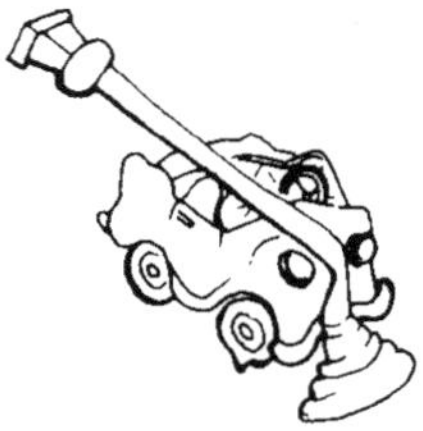

destruction

****

236 -<u>rrhagia</u> is the suffix meaning excessive flow or discharge. Thus, hemor<u>rhage</u> is a term meaning __________ of blood.

hem'or-ij

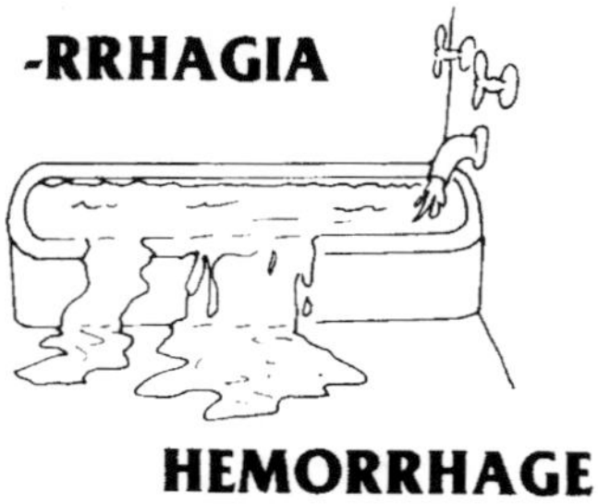

excessive flow/discharge

****

237 Another suffix meaning excessive discharge or flow is -<u>rrhea</u>. Dia<u>rrhea</u> is the medical term for __________ __________ of the bowel.

di"ah-re'ah

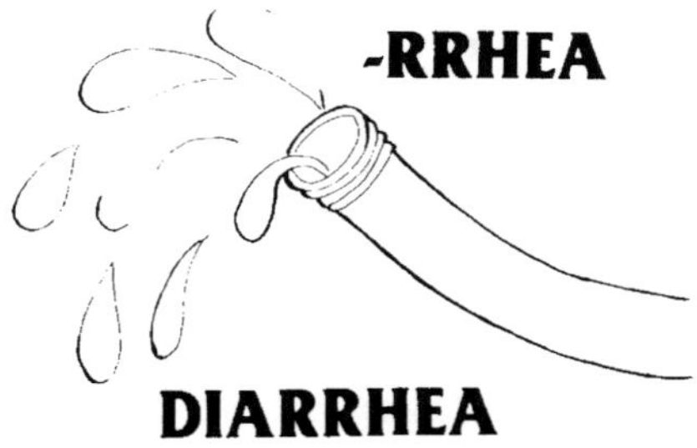

excessive discharge

****

238 -<u>penia</u> is the suffix meaning decrease or deficiency. Erythro<u>penia</u> means a __________ of red blood cells.

e-rith"ro-pe'ne-ah

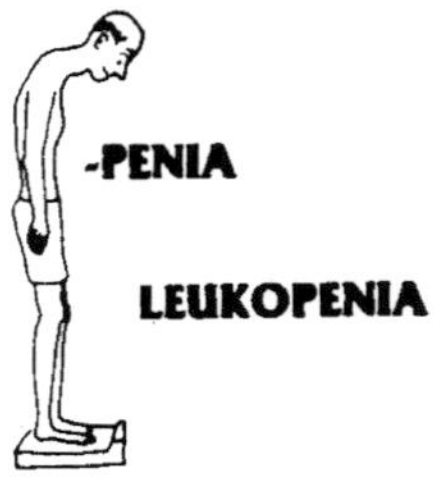

deficiency/decrease

****

239 -<u>spasm</u> is the suffix meaning involuntary contraction. The medical term myo<u>spasm</u>, then, means an __________ __________ of the muscle.

mi'o-spazm

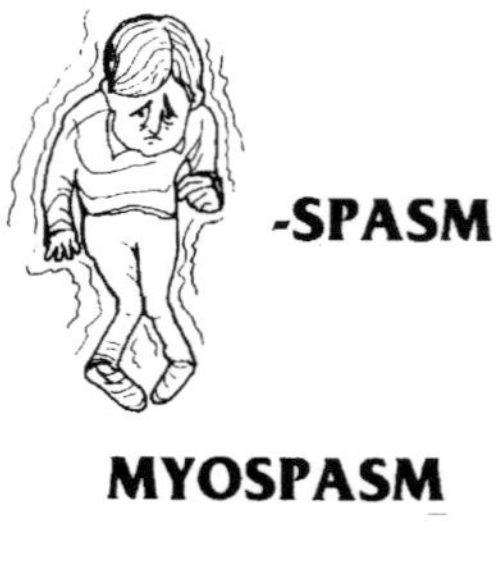

involuntary contraction

****

240 The suffixes -ic, -ac, -al, and -ar mean pertaining to. Cardiovascular, for example, means __________ __________ the heart and vessels.

kar"de-o-vas'ku-lar

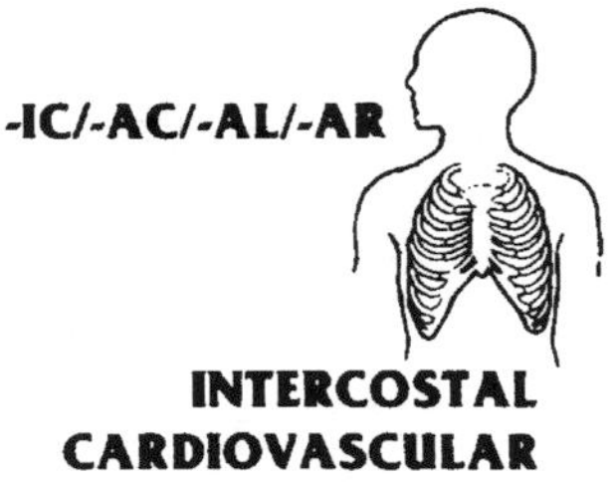

pertaining to

****

241 Here's another example: Intercostal means __________ __________ between the ribs.

in"ter-kos'tal

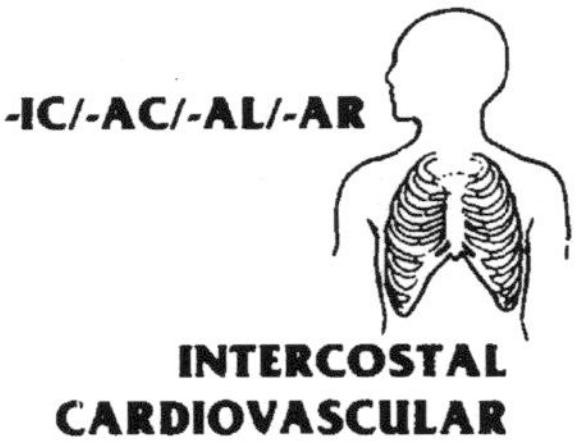

pertaining to

****

242 Otoscopic means __________ __________ an examination of the ear.

o'to-skop-ik

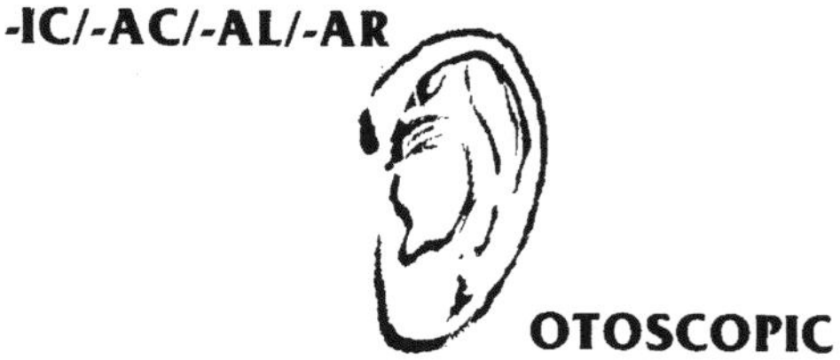

pertaining to

****

243 Finally, cardiac means __________ __________ the heart.

kar'de-ak

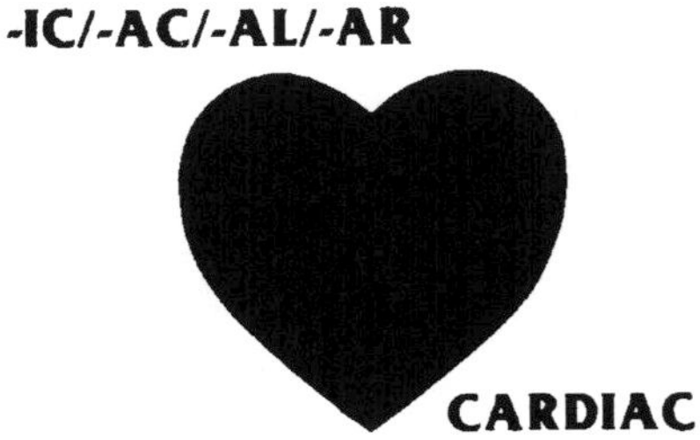

pertaining to

****

244 In review, write the meaning of each of the following symptomatic suffixes:

a. -algia means: ___________

pain (frame 233)

****

b. -genic means: ___________

producing (frame 234)

****

c. -lysis means: ___________

destruction (frame 235)

****

d. -rrhagia means: ___________

excessive discharge/flow (frame 236)

****

e. -rrhea means: ___________

excessive discharge (frame 237)

****

f. -penia means: ___________

deficiency (frame 238)

****

g. -ic, -ac, -al, and -ar mean: ___________

pertaining to (frame 240)

****

h. -spasm means: ___________

involuntary contraction (frame 239)

****

245 To further reinforce what you have learned, please write the correct word in the blanks in the following sentences.

a. Dentalgia is the medical term for a ___________ in the tooth.

pain (frame 233)

****

b. Pyogenic is the term for __________ pus.

producing (frame 234)

****

c. Hemolysis means the _________ of red blood cells.

destruction (frame 235)

****

d. Hemorrhage is a term meaning __________ of blood.

excessive discharge/flow (frame 236)

****

e. Erythropenia means a __________ of red blood cells.

deficiency (frame 237)

****

f. Diarrhea is the medical term for __________ __________ of the bowel.

excessive discharge (frame 238)

****

g. Myospasm is the medical term for __________ __________ of a muscle.

involuntary contraction (frame 239)

****

h. Cardiovascular means _________ __________ the heart and vessels.

pertaining to (frame 240)

****

i. Intercostal means __________ __________ between the ribs.

pertaining to (frame 241)

****

j. Otoscopic means __________ __________ an examination of the ear.

pertaining to (frame 242)

****

k. Cardiac means __________ __________ the heart.

pertaining to (frame 243)

****

If you missed any of the questions in frames 244 and 245, please review the appropriate frame(s) before continuing.

CONGRATULATIONS

You have completed the last lesson on medical terminology. With your knowledge of prefixes, stems, and suffixes, you should be able to recognize and define most medical terms.

****

Continue with Self-Assessment

Section VI. SELF-ASSESSMENT #3

You have now completed lesson 4. To evaluate how well you have learned the suffixes covered in lesson 4, complete the self-assessment #3 questions. This self-assessment is to assist you in determining whether you need to go back and review parts of lesson 4 before going to self-assessment #4 which is an exercise covering all stems, prefixes, and suffixes you have studied in this course.

SELF-ASSESSMENT #3

SUFFIXES

LISTED BELOW IN COLUMN "A" ARE 10 OF THE 35 LATIN AND GREEK STEMS GIVEN TO YOU. IN COLUMN "B" ARE THE ENGLISH MEANINGS OF THESE SUFFIXES. MATCH THE TWO, AND WRITE THE ENGLISH MEANING FROM COLUMN "B" NEXT TO THE NUMBER IN COLUMN "A."

EXAMPLE: EMIA = BLOOD

COLUMN A			COLUMN B
1.	_____________ SCLEROSIS	A.	INFLAMMATION
2.	_____________ PTOSIS	B.	PLASTIC REPAIR
3.	_____________ TROPHY	C.	INVOLUNTARY CONTRACTION
4.	_____________ ITIS	D.	OPENING/INCISION INTO
5.	_____________ MEGALY	E.	HARDENING
6.	_____________ PLASTY	F.	TUMOR
7.	_____________ TOMY	G.	GROWTH/NOURISHMENT
8.	_____________ OMA	H.	DOWNWARD DISPLACEMENT
9.	_____________ ALGIA	I.	ENLARGEMENT
10.	_____________ SPASM	J.	PAIN/ACHE

SELF-ASSESSMENT QUIZ #3

SUFFIXES

FOR EACH OF THE MULTIPLE CHOICE QUESTIONS BELOW, SELECT THE ONE MOST APPROPRIATE ANSWER. CIRCLE THE ANSWER.

11. THE SUFFIX -OSIS IN THE WORD DERMATOPHYTOSIS MEANS:

    A. GROWING
    B. CONDITION
    C. DROOPING
    D. DILATION

12. THE SUFFIX -MEGALY IN THE WORD HEPATOSPLENOMEGALY MEANS:

    A. SOFTENING
    B. HARDENING
    C. ENLARGEMENT
    D. SWELLING

13. THE SUFFIX -IASIS IN THE WORD NEPHROLITHIASIS MEANS:

    A. CONDITION/PRESENCE OF
    B. GROWTH/NOURISHMENT
    C. SUSPENSION/FIXATION
    D. PROTRUSION/SWELLING

14. THE SUFFIX -ECTOMY IN THE WORD SALPINGO-OOPHORECTOMY MEANS:

    A. EXCISION OF
    B. OPENING OF
    C. INSPECTION OF
    D. SUSPENSION OF

15. THE SUFFIX -IC IN THE WORD OTOSCOPIC MEANS:

    A. REPAIR OF
    B. SOFTENING OF
    C. CONDITION OF
    D. PERTAINING TO

16. THE SUFFIX -CENTESIS IN THE WORD ARTHROCENTESIS MEANS:

    A. DESTRUCTION OF
    B. PUNCTURE OF
    C. PERTAINING TO
    D. ORIGINATING IN

17. THE SUFFIX -MALACIA IN THE WORD CHONDROMALACIA MEANS:

    A. HARDENING
    B. SOFTENING
    C. FLOWING
    D. PRODUCING

SELF-ASSESSMENT QUIZ #3

SUFFIXES

18. THE SUFFIX -DESIS IN THE WORD ARTHRODESIS MEANS:

    A. FIXATION
    B. DILATION
    C. PUNCTURE
    D. ENLARGEMENT

19. THE SUFFIX -AR IN THE WORD CARDIOVASCULAR MEANS:

    A. PERTAINING TO
    B. INSPECTION OF
    C. SOFTENING OF
    D. NOURISHMENT OF

20. THE SUFFIX -PHOBIA IN THE WORD HYDROPHOBIA MEANS:

    A. OPENING OF
    B. LIKE OF
    C. DISEASE OF
    D. FEAR OF

Check your answers on the following pages

SOLUTIONS FOR SELF-ASSESSMENT #3

SUFFIXES

1. E (HARDENING) SCLEROSIS
2. H (DOWNWARD DISPLACEMENT) PTOSIS
3. G (GROWTH/NOURISHMENT) TROPHY
4. A (INFLAMMATION) ITIS
5. I (ENLARGEMENT) MEGALY
6. B (PLASTIC REPAIR) PLASTY
7. D (OPENING/INCISION INTO) TOMY
8. F (TUMOR) OMA
9. J (PAIN/ACHE) ALGIA
10. C (INVOLUNTARY CONTRACTION) SPASM

SOLUTIONS FOR SELF-ASSESSMENT QUIZ #3

SUFFIXES

11. THE SUFFIX -"OSIS" IN THE WORD DERMATOPHYTOSIS MEANS:

    B. CONDITION

12. THE SUFFIX -"MEGALY" IN THE WORD HEPATOSPLENOMEGALY MEANS:

    C. ENLARGEMENT

13. THE SUFFIX -"IASIS" IN THE WORD NEPHROLITHIASIS MEANS:

    A. CONDITION/PRESENCE OF

14. THE SUFFIX -"ECTOMY" IN THE WORD SALPINGO-OOPHORECTOMY MEANS:

    A. EXCISION OF

15. THE SUFFIX -"IC" IN THE WORD OTOSCOPIC MEANS:

    D. PERTAINING TO

16. THE SUFFIX -"CENTESIS" IN THE WORD ARTHROCENTESIS MEANS:

    B. PUNCTURE OF

17. THE SUFFIX -"MALACIA" IN THE WORD CHONDROMALACIA MEANS:

    B. SOFTENING

18. THE SUFFIX -"DESIS" IN THE WORD ARTHRODESIS MEANS:

    A. FIXATION

19. THE SUFFIX -"AR" IN THE WORD CARDIOVASCULAR MEANS:

    A. PERTAINING TO

20. THE SUFFIX -"PHOBIA" IN THE WORD HYDROPHOBIA MEANS:

    D. FEAR OF

Continue with Self-Assessment #4 (Review)

SOLUTIONS TO PRETEST #3

1. Disease
2. Hemorrhage
3. Hardening
4. Softening
5. Breakdown (destruction)
6. Dilatation
7. Pain
8. Blood
9. Hernia
10. Condition
11. Tumor
12. Inflammation
13. Puncture
14. Discharge
15. Surgical repair/plastic repair
16. Decrease/deficiency
17. Fixation/suspension
18. Incision
19. Opening
20. Examination
21. Suturing
22. Prolapse
23. Fear
24. Enlarged
25. Dilatation
26. Overdevelopment/enlargement
27. Removal
28. Rupture

Continue with Lesson 4

REVIEW - SELF-ASSESSMENT #4

You have completed all the study material on medical terminology. Self-assessment #4 is a review of all the material you have been given. It consists of 78 Latin or Greek medical terms composed of the prefixes, stems, and suffixes you have studied. You are required to match the English meaning of the terms with the Latin or Greek term.

EXAMPLE

COLUMN A	COLUMN B
1. ________ Inflammation of the bones and joints.	A. OSTEOARTHRITIS

SELF-ASSESSMENT #4

MEDICAL TERMS

This quiz is a review of all the material you have been given. Column "A" contains the meanings of the medical terms, and column "B" contains the Latin or Greek term composed of the prefixes, stems, and suffixes you have studied. Match column "A" with column "B." Enter the letter of the medical term in the space provided. All matching terms are on the same page.

		COLUMN A	COLUMN B
1.	___	Condition of stones in the kidney	A. Dyspnea
2.	___	Inflammation of many nerves	B. Nocturia
3.	___	Excessive vomiting	C. Afebrile
4.	___	Inflammation of the stomach and intestine	D. Oliguria
5.	___	Tumor of the brain.	E. Cerebroma
6.	___	Inflammation of the liver	F. Hyperemesis
7.	___	Scant urine	G. Hematoma
8.	___	Without fever	H. Salpingitis
9.	___	Under the skin	I. Duodenal
10.	___	Inside the abdomen	J. Chondritis
11.	___	Night urine	K. Gastroenteritis
12.	___	Involuntary contraction of a muscle	L. Nephrolithiasis
13.	___	Difficult breathing	M. Hepatitis
14.	___	Inflammation of the cartilage	N. Myospasm
15.	___	Pertaining to first part of small intestine	O. Subcutaneous
16.	___	Tumor filled with blood	P. Glucosuria
17.	___	Sugar in the urine	Q. Intra-abdominal
18.	___	Inflammation of the tubes	R. Polyneuritis

SELF-ASSESSMENT #4 (Part 2)

		COLUMN A		COLUMN B
1.	___	Inflammation within the uterus	A.	Arthrocentesis
2.	___	Removal of both tubes and ovaries	B.	Hysterectomy
3.	___	Suture repair of a hernia	C.	Adenectomy
4.	___	Fixation of the testes	D.	Laparotomy
5.	___	Suture repair of the tongue	E.	Arthrodesis
6.	___	Removal of a kidney	F.	Laryngoscope
7.	___	Removal of the stomach	G.	Otoplasty
8.	___	Artificial opening into the colon	H.	Gastrectomy
9.	___	Plastic repair of the ear	I.	Glossorrhaphy
10.	___	Plastic repair of the nose	J.	Endometritis
11.	___	Instrument used for examination of the larynx	K.	Tympanoplasty
12.	___	Plastic operation upon the lip	L.	Herniorrhaphy
13.	___	Surgical fixation of a joint	M.	Cholecystectomy
14.	___	Puncture of the thorax	N.	Colostomy
15.	___	Incision into the abdominal wall	O.	Bilateral Salpingo-oophorectomy
16.	___	Plastic repair of the eardrum	P.	Cheiloplasty
17.	___	Removal of a gland	Q.	Orchiopexy
18.	___	Removal of the uterus	R.	Nephrectomy
19.	___	Removal of the gallbladder	S.	Rhinoplasty
20.	___	Puncture of a joint for removal of fluid	T.	Thoracentesis

SELF-ASSESSMENT #4 (Part 3)

		COLUMN A		COLUMN B
1.	___	Hardening of the arteries	A.	Hepatosplenomegaly
2.	___	Inflammation of the tongue	B.	Hypertrophy
3.	___	Downward displacement of the eyelids	C.	Monocyte
4.	___	Condition of blueness	D.	Thrombophlebitis
5.	___	Pertaining to the heart and vessels	E.	Otoscopic
6.	___	Between the ribs	F.	Lipoma
7.	___	Fear of water	G.	Polyphagia
8.	___	Condition of fungus of the skin	H.	Tachycardia
9.	___	Inflammation of the bones and joints	I.	Bradycardia
10.	___	Fast heart beat	J.	Anesthesia
11.	___	Slow heart beat	K.	Hydrophobia
12.	___	Without feeling or sensation	L.	Arteriosclerosis
13.	___	Pertaining to examination of the ear	M.	Cardiovascular
14.	___	Inflammation of a vein with a clot	N.	Blepharoptosis
15.	___	Enlargement of the liver and spleen	O.	Glossitis
16.	___	Fatty tumor	P.	Osteoarthritis
17.	___	Excessive growth	Q.	Cyanosis
18.	___	Red cell	R.	Intercostal
19.	___	Single or one cell	S.	Erythrocyte
20.	___	Excessive eating	T.	Dermatophytosis

SELF-ASSESSMENT #4 (Part 4)

		COLUMN A		COLUMN B
1.	___	Suspension of testes	A.	Hypotension
2.	___	Enlargement of the kidney	B.	Encephalitis
3.	___	Inflammation of the cornea	C.	Dentalgia
4.	___	Producing pus	D.	Cystitis
5.	___	Condition of dead tissue	E.	Hematuria
6.	___	Softening of the cartilage	F.	Myalgia
7.	___	Pertaining to the liver	G.	Hematemesis
8.	___	Vomiting of blood	H.	Pericarditis
9.	___	Inflammation of the nose	I.	Necrosis
10.	___	Blood in the urine	J.	Nephromegaly
11.	___	Inflammation within the heart	K.	Orchiopexy
12.	___	Resembling a gland	L.	Keratitis
13.	___	Pain in a muscle	M.	Pyogenic
14.	___	Low blood pressure	N.	Hepatic
15.	___	High blood pressure	O.	Chondromalacia
16.	___	Inflammation of the brain	P.	Acromegaly
17.	___	Inflammation around the heart	Q.	Hypertension
18.	___	Tooth ache/pain	R.	Endocarditis
19.	___	Enlargement of the extremities	S.	Adenoid
20.	___	Inflammation of the bladder	T.	Rhinitis

Check your answers on the following pages

SOLUTIONS FOR SELF-ASSESSMENT #4

MEDICAL TERMS

		COLUMN A		COLUMN B
1.	L	Condition of stones in the kidney	A.	Dyspnea
2.	R	Inflammation of many nerves	B.	Nocturia
3.	F	Excessive vomiting	C.	Afebrile
4.	K	Inflammation of the stomach and intestine	D.	Oliguria
5.	E	Tumor of the brain.	E.	Cerebroma
6.	M	Inflammation of the liver	F.	Hyperemesis
7.	D	Scant urine	G.	Hematoma
8.	C	Without fever	H.	Salpingitis
9.	O	Under the skin	I.	Duodenal
10.	Q	Inside the abdomen	J.	Chondritis
11.	B	Night urine	K.	Gastroenteritis
12.	N	Involuntary contraction of a muscle	L.	Nephrolithiasis
13.	A	Difficult breathing	M.	Hepatitis
14.	J	Inflammation of the cartilage	N.	Myospasm
15.	I	Pertaining to first part of small intestine	O.	Subcutaneous
16.	G	Tumor filled with blood	P.	Glucosuria
17.	P	Sugar in the urine	Q.	Intra-abdominal
18.	H	Inflammation of the tubes	R.	Polyneuritis

SOLUTIONS FOR SELF-ASSESSMENT #4 (Part 2)

	COLUMN A			COLUMN B
1.	J	Inflammation within the uterus	A.	Arthrocentesis
2.	O	Removal of both tubes and ovaries	B.	Hysterectomy
3.	L	Suture repair of a hernia	C.	Adenectomy
4.	Q	Fixation of the testes	D.	Laparotomy
5.	I	Suture repair of the tongue	E.	Arthrodesis
6.	R	Removal of a kidney	F.	Laryngoscope
7.	H	Removal of the stomach	G.	Otoplasty
8.	N	Artificial opening into the colon	H.	Gastrectomy
9.	G	Plastic repair of the ears	I.	Glossorrhaphy
10.	S	Plastic repair of the nose	J.	Endometritis
11.	F	Instrument used for examination of the larynx	K.	Tympanoplasty
12.	P	Plastic operation upon the lip	L.	Herniorrhaphy
13.	E	Surgical fixation of a joint	M.	Cholecystectomy
14.	T	Puncture of the thorax	N.	Colostomy
15.	D	Incision into the abdominal wall	O.	Bilateral Salpingo-oophorectomy
16.	K	Plastic repair of the eardrum	P.	Cheiloplasty
17.	C	Removal of a gland	Q.	Orchiopexy
18.	B	Removal of the uterus	R.	Nephrectomy
19.	M	Removal of the gallbladder	S.	Rhinoplasty
20.	A	Puncture of a joint for removal of fluid	T.	Thoracentesis

SOLUTIONS FOR SELF-ASSESSMENT #4 (Part 3)

	Answer	COLUMN A		COLUMN B
1.	L	Hardening of the arteries	A.	Hepatosplenomegaly
2.	O	Inflammation of the tongue	B.	Hypertrophy
3.	N	Downward displacement of the eyelids	C.	Monocyte
4.	Q	Condition of blueness	D.	Thrombophlebitis
5.	M	Pertaining to the heart and vessels	E.	Otoscopic
6.	R	Between the ribs	F.	Lipoma
7.	K	Fear of water	G.	Polyphagia
8.	T	Condition of fungus of the skin	H.	Tachycardia
9.	P	Inflammation of the bones and joints	I.	Bradycardia
10.	H	Fast heart beat	J.	Anesthesia
11.	I	Slow heart beat	K.	Hydrophobia
12.	J	Without feeling or sensation	L.	Arteriosclerosis
13.	E	Pertaining to examination of the ear	M.	Cardiovascular
14.	D	Inflammation of a vein with a clot	N.	Blepharoptosis
15.	A	Enlargement of the liver and spleen	O.	Glossitis
16.	F	Fatty tumor	P.	Osteoarthritis
17.	B	Excessive growth	Q.	Cyanosis
18.	S	Red cell	R.	Intercostal
19.	C	Single or one cell	S.	Erythrocyte
20.	G	Excessive eating	T.	Dermatophytosis

SOLUTIONS FOR SELF-ASSESSMENT #4 (Part 4)

	Answer	COLUMN A		COLUMN B
1.	K	Suspension of testes	A.	Hypotension
2.	J	Enlargement of the kidney	B.	Encephalitis
3.	L	Inflammation of the cornea	C.	Dentalgia
4.	M	Producing pus	D.	Cystitis
5.	I	Condition of dead tissue	E.	Hematuria
6.	O	Softening of the cartilage	F.	Myalgia
7.	N	Pertaining to the liver	G.	Hematemesis
8.	G	Vomiting of blood	H.	Pericarditis
9.	T	Inflammation of the nose	I.	Necrosis
10.	E	Blood in the urine	J.	Nephromegaly
11.	R	Inflammation within the heart	K.	Orchiopexy
12.	S	Resembling a gland	L.	Keratitis
13.	F	Pain in a muscle	M.	Pyogenic
14.	A	Low blood pressure	N.	Hepatic
15.	Q	High blood pressure	O.	Chondromalacia
16.	B	Inflammation of the brain	P.	Acromegaly
17.	H	Inflammation around the heart	Q.	Hypertension
18.	C	Tooth ache/pain	R.	Endocarditis
19.	P	Enlargement of the extremities	S.	Adenoid
20.	D	Inflammation of the bladder	T.	Rhinitis

GLOSSARY

Medical Term	Meaning
A	
Acromegaly	Enlargement of the extremities
Adenoid	Resembling a gland
Afebrile	Without fever
Anesthesia	Without feeling or sensation
Arteriosclerosis	Hardening of the arteries
B	
Blepharoptosis	Downward displacement of the eyelids
Bradycardia	Slow heartbeat
C	
Cardiovascular	Pertaining to the heart and vessels
Cerebroma	Tumor of the brain
Chondritis	Inflammation of the cartilage
Chondromalacia	Softening of the cartilage
Cyanosis.	Condition of blueness
Cystitis	Inflammation of the bladder
D	
Dentalgia	Toothache/pain
Dermatophytosis	Condition of fungus of the skin
Duodenal	Pertaining to the first part of small intestine
Dyspnea	Difficult breathing
E	
Encephalitis	Inflammation of the brain
Endocarditis	Inflammation within the heart
Endometritis	Inflammation within the uterus
Erythrocyte	Red cell

Medical Term	Meaning
G	
Gastroenteritis	Inflammation of the stomach and intestine
Glossitis	Inflammation of the tongue
Glucosuria	Sugar in the urine
H	
Hematemesis	.Vomiting of blood
Hematoma	Tumor filled with blood
Hematuria	Blood in the urine
Hepatic	Pertaining to the liver
Hepatitis	Inflammation of the liver
Hepatosplenomegaly	Enlargement of the liver and spleen
Hydrophobia	Fear of water
Hyperemesis	.Excessive vomiting
Hypertension	High blood pressure
Hypertrophy	Excessive growth
Hypotension	Low blood pressure
I	
Intercostal	Between the ribs
Intra-Abdominal	Inside the abdomen
K	
Keratitis	Inflammation of the cornea
L	
Lipoma	Fatty tumor

Medical Term	Meaning
M	
Monocyte	Single or one cell
Myalgia	Pain in the muscle
Myospasm	Involuntary contraction of a muscle
N	
Necrosis	Condition of dead tissue
Nephrolithiasis	Condition of stones in the kidney
Nephrolithiasis	Enlargement of the kidney
Nocturia	Night urine
O	
Oliguria	Scant urine
Osteoarthritis	Inflammation of the bones and joints
Otoscopic	Pertaining to examination of the ear
P	
Pericarditis	Inflammation around the heart
Polyneuritis	Inflammation of many nerves
Polyphagia	Excessive eating
Postpartum	After birth
Pyogenic	Producing pus
R	
Rhinitis	Inflammation of the nose
S	
Salpingitis	Inflammation of the tubes

Medical Term	Meaning
T	
Tachycardia	Fast heartbeat
Thrombophlebitis	Inflammation of a vein with a clot

Operations or Procedures	Meaning
Adenectomy	Removal of a gland
Arthrocentesis	Puncture of a joint for removal of fluid
Arthrodesis	Surgical fixation of a joint
Cheiloplasty	Plastic operation upon the lip
Cholecystectomy	Removal of the gallbladder
Colostomy	Incision into the colon
Gastrectomy	Removal of the stomach
Glossorrhaphy	Suture repair of the tongue
Herniorrhaphy	Suture repair of a hernia
Hysterectomy	Removal of the uterus
Laparotomy	Incision into the abdominal wall
Laryngoscopy	Examination of the larynx with an instrument
Nephrectomy	Removal of a kidney
Orchiopexy	Fixation of the testes
Otoplasty	Plastic repair of the ears
Rhinoplasty	Plastic repair of the nose
Thoracentesis	Puncture of the thorax
Tympanoplasty	Plastic repair of the eardrum

PRONUNCIATION GUIDE FOR MEDICAL TERMS USED IN LESSON 2

USE THIS GUIDE TO ASSIST YOU IN PRONUNCIATION

IF IT IS AN	AND	THEN IT IS
UNMARKED VOWEL	IT ENDS A SYLLABLE	LONG "ā" (UNLESS OTHERWISE INDICATED)
	THE SYLLABLE ENDS IN A CONSONANT	SHORT "ă" (UNLESS OTHERWISE INDICATED)

MEDICAL TERM

Abdominal /ab-dom'i-nal/

Acrodermatitis /ak"ro-der"mah-ti'tis/

Acromegaly /ak"ro-meg' ah-le/

Adenectomy /ad"e-nek' to-me/

Afebrile /a-feb' ril/

Anesthesia /an"es-the'ze-ah/

Angiogram /an'je-o-gram"/

Arteriosclerosis/ar-te"re-o-skle'ro'sis/

Arthrodesis /ar"thro-de'sis/

Blepharitis /blef"ah-ri'tis/

Bronchitis /brong-ki'tis/

Cardiovascular /kar"de-o-vas'ku-lar/

Celiectomy / se"le-ek'to-me/

Cheiloplasty /ki'lo-plas"te/

Chondritis /kon-dri'tis/

Cholecystectomy /ko"le-sis-tek'to-me/

Colon /ko'lon/

Colostomy /ko'los'to-me/

Cystitis /sis-ti'tis/

Dacryocystitis /dak"re-o-sis-ti'tis/

Dentalgia /den'tal'je-ah/

Duodenal /du'o-de'nal/

Endometritis /en"do-me"tri'tis/

Encephalitis /en"sef-ah-li'tis/

Erythrocyte /e-rith'ro-sit/

Gastrectomy /gas-trek'to-me/

Gastroenteritis /gas"tro-en-ter-i'tis/

Gingivitis /jin"ji-vi'tis/

Glossitis /glos-si'tis/

Glucosuria /gloo"ko-su're-ah/

Hematology /hem"ah tol'o-je/

Hematoma /hem"ah-to'mah/

Hepatitis /hep"ah-ti'tis/

Hydrophobia /hi"dro-fo'be-ah/

Hyperemesis /hi"per-em'e-sis/

Hysterectomy /his"te-rek'to-me/

Ileitis /il"e-i'tis/

Ileum /il'e-um/

Intercostal /in"ter-kos'tal/

Jejunum /je-joo'num/

Jejunectomy /je"joo-nek'to-me/

Keratitis /ker"ah-ti'tis/

Laparotomy /lap-ah-rot'o-me/

Laryngoscopy/lar"ing-gos'ko-pe/

Lingual /ling'gwal/

Lipoma /li-po mah/

Lymphocyte /lim'fo-sit/

Mycosis /mi-ko'sis/

Myelitis /mi"e-li'tis/

Myospasm /mi'o-spazm/

Myringotomy /mir"in-got'o-me/

Necropsy /nek'rop-se/

Nephrectomy /ne-frek'to-me/

Nephrolithiasis/nef"ro-li-thi'ah-sis/

Nocturia /nok-tu're-ah/

Ocular /ok'u-lar/

Onychectomy /on"i-kek'-to-me/

Oophorectomy /o"of-o-rek'to-me/

Ophthalmology /of"thal- mol' o-je/

Optometrist /op-tom'e-trist/

Orchiopexy /or"ke-o-pek'se/

Osteoarthritis /os"te-o-ar-thri'-tis/

Otoplasty /o'to-plas"te/

Phagocyte /fag'o-sit/

Phlebectomy /fle-bek'to-me/

Pneodynamics /ne'o-di-nam'iks/

Pneumonia /nu-mo'ne-ah/

Pneumatic /nu-mat-ik/

Polyneuritis /pol"e-nu-ri'tis/

Polyphagia /pol"e-fa'je-ah/

Proctitis /prok-ti'tis/

Psychology /si-kol 'o-je/

Pulmonary /pul'mo-ner"e/

Pyogenic /pi"o-jen'ik/

Pyromania /pi"ro-ma'ne-ah/

Rhinitis /ri-ni'tis/

Salpingitis /sal"pin-ji'tis/

Splenectomy /sple-nek'to-me/

Stomatitis /sto-mah-ti'tis/

Tendinitis /ten"di-ni'tis/

Thrombophlebitis /throm"bo-fle-bi'tis

Tinea Pedis /tin'e-ah/ Pe'dis/

Tracheitis /tra"ke-i'tis/

Tympanoplasty /tim"pah-no-plas'te/

Ureteritis /u"re-ter-i'tis/

Urethritis /u"re-thri'tis/

Vasodilator /vas"o-di-lat'or/

Venogram /ve'no-gram/

PRONUNCIATION GUIDE FOR
MEDICAL TERMS USED IN LESSON 3

MEDICAL TERM

Afebrile /a-feb'ril/

Anesthesia /an"es-the'ze-ah/

Antepartum /an'te-par'tum/

Antitoxin /an"ti-tok'sin/

Anterolateral /an"ter-o-lat'er-al/

Bilateral /bi-lat'er-al/

Bradycardia /brad"e-kar'de-ah/

Cyanosis /si"ah-no'sis/

Dextrocardia /deks"tro-kar'de-ah/

Dyspnea /disp'ne-ah/

Ectopic /ek-top'ik/

Empyema /em"pi-e'mah/

Endometritis /en"do-me-tri'tis/

Erythrocyte /e-rith'ro-sit/

Hemiplegia /hem"e-ple'je-ah/

Hydrophobia /hi"dro-fo'be-ah/

Hyperemesis /hi"per-em'e-sis/

Hypertension /hi"per-ten'shun/

Hypodermic /hi"po-der'mik/

Hypotension /hi"po-ten'shun/

Intercostal /in"ter-kos'tal/

Intra-abdominal /in"trah-ab-dom'i-nal/

Leukocyte /lu'ko-sit/

Levoversion /le"vo-ver'zhun/

Macroscopic /mak"ro-skop'ik/

Macrocyte /mak'ro-sit/

Malodorous /mal-o der-es/

Medial /me'de-al/

Megacolon /meg"ah-ko'lon/

Melanoma /mel"ah-no'mah/

Microcardia/mi"kro-kar'de-ah/

Microcyte /mi'kro-sit/

Monocyte /mon'o-sit/

Multipara /mul-tip'ah-rah/

Nocturia /nok-ru're-ah/

Oliguria /ol"i gu're-ah/

Panhysterectomy /pan"his-ter-ek'to-me/

Pericarditis /per"i-kar-di-tis/

Postoperative /post-op'er-a"tiv/

Postnasal /post-na'zal/

Polyneuritis /pol"e-nu-ri'tis/

Posterolateral /pos"ter-o-lat'er-al/

Preoperative /pre-op'er-a"tiv/

Quadriplegia /kwod"ri-ple' je-ah/

Retrocardial /ret"ro-kar'de-al/

Semiconscious /sem"e-kon'shus/

Subcutaneous /sub"ku-ta'ne-us/

Tachycardia /tak"e-kar'de-ah/

Tricuspid /tri-kus'pid/

PRONUNCIATION GUIDE FOR
MEDICAL TERMS USED IN LESSON 4

MEDICAL TERM

Acromegaly /ak"ro-meg'ah-le/

Angiectasis /an"je-ek'tah-sis/

Arteriosclerosis/ar-te"re-o-skle'ro'sis/

Arthrocentesis /ar"thro-sen-te'sis/

Arthrodesis /ar"thro-de'sis/

Blepharoptosis /blef"ah-ro-to'sis/

Bronchogenic /brong-ko-jen'ik/

Bronchoscopy /brong-kos'ko-pe/

Cardiac /kar'de-ak'/

Cardiorrhexis /kar"de-o-rek'sis/

Cardiovascular /kar"de-o-vas'ku-lar/

Cholecystectomy /ko"le-sis-tek'to-me/

Cholelithiasis /ko"le-li-thi'ah-sis/

Chondritis /kon-dri'tis/

Chondromalacia / kon"dro-mah-la'she-ah/

Colostomy /ko'los'to-me/

Cyanosis /si"ah-no'sis/

Dentalgia /den'tal'je-ah/

Dermatophytosis /der"mah-to-fi-to'sis/

Diarrhea /di"ah-re'ah/

Encephalitis /en"sef-ah-li'tis/

Enterolysis /en"ter-ol i-sis/

Erythropenia /e-rith"ro-pe'ne-ah/

Gastrocele /gas'tro-sel/

Hematoma /hem"ah-to'mah/

Hemorrhage /hem'or-ij/

Hepatoma /hep"ah-to'mah/

Hepatosplenomegaly

/hep"ah-to-sple"no-meg'ah-le/

Hydroarthrosis /hi"dro-ar" thro'sis/

Hydrophobia /hi"dro-fo'be-ah/

Hypertrophy /hi-per'tro-fe/

Hypoglycemia /hi"po-gli-s 'me-ah e/

Intercostal in"ter-kos'tal/

Laparotomy /lap-ah-rot'o-me/

Leukemia /lu-ke'me-ah/

Leukopenia /lu"ko-pe'ne-ah/

Lipoma /li-po mah/

Lymphadenopathy /lim-fad"e-nop' ah-the/

Myocarditis /mi"o-kar-di'tis/

Myocardium /mi"o-kar'de-um/

Myospasm /mi"o-spazm/

Nephrolithiasis /nef"ro-li- thi'ah-sis/

Neuropathy /nu-rop'ah-the/

Neurorrhaphy /nu-ror'ah-fe/

Orchiopexy /or"ke-o-pek'se/

Otoscopic /o'to-skop-ik/

Pyogenic /pi"o-jen'ik/

Psychogenic /si"ko-jen'ik/

Rhinoplasty /ri no-plas"te/

Salpingo-oophorectomy

/sal-ping"go-o"of-o-rek'to-me/

Subhepatic /sub"he-pat'ik/

Tympanoplasty /tim"pah-no- plas'te/

MEDICAL ABBREVIATIONS AND SYMBOLS

This appendix is a list of commonly used medical abbreviations and symbols which are authorized to be used in medical records. (For a complete list of authorized medical abbreviations and symbols, see AR 40-66.)

A; a	before
AAE	acute allergic encephalitis
Ab	antibodies
abd hyst	abdominal hysterectomy
ABE	acute bacterial endocarditis
ABP	arterial blood pressure
ABR	absolute bed rest
ABS	acute brain syndrome
ac	before meals
ACA	adenocarcinoma
ACH	acetylcholine
ACI	adrenal cortical insufficiency
ACTH	adrenocorticotropic hormone
ACVD	acute cardiovascular disease
AD	right ear
A & D	admission and discharge
ADD	average daily dose
adhib	to be administered
ADL	activities of daily living
ad lib	as desired
adm	admission; admit; admitted
ADS	antibody deficiency syndrome
AE	above the elbow
AF	acid-fast

AFB	acid-fast bacilli
afeb	afebrile; without fever
AF/F	atrial fibrillation and/or flutter
AGG	agammaglobulinemia
AHAC	American Heart Association Classification
AHD	atherosclerotic heart disease
AI	aortic insufficiency or incompetence
AID	acute infectious disease
AIHA	autoimmune hemolytic anemia
AJ	ankle jerk
AK amp	above the knee amputation
ALMI	anterior lateral myocardial infarct
alt die (dieb)	alternate days; every other night
alt noc (noct)	alternate nights; every other night
ALVF	acute left ventricular failure
AMA	against medical advice
amb	ambulatory
AMI	acute myocardial infarction
anti-HAA	antibody hepatitis-associated antigen
AOB	alcohol on breath
ap	before dinner
A & P	anterior and posterior
APB	atrial or auricular premature beat
APC	aspirin (acetylsalicylic acid), phenacetin, caffeine
aq	water
AS	left ear
ASA	acetylsalicylic acid (aspirin)
ASAP	as soon as possible

ASHD	arteriosclerotic heart disease
ASS	anterior superior spine
A-S syndrome	Adams-Stokes syndrome
AU	both ears
ax	axillary
B	born
BA	blood alcohol
B/A	backache
BBB	bundle branch block
BC	bone conduction
BCP	birth control pills
BE	barium enema
BH	bundle of His
bib	drink
bid	twice a day
bin	twice during the night
B/J; B&J	bone and joint
BM	bowel movement
BMR	basal metabolic rate
bol	pill
BOM	bilateral otitis media
BP	blood pressure
BPH	benign prostatic hypertrophy
BPI	blood pressure increased
BS	bowel or breath sound(s)
BSO	bilateral salpingo-oophorectomy
BTL	bilateral tubal ligation
BUE	both upper extremities

BUN	blood urea nitrogen
BUQ	both upper quadrants
BV	blood volume
BW	body weight
Bx	biopsy
C1 to C7	cervical nerves or vertebrae 1 to 7
CI to CXII	cranial nerves
c	with
CA	cardiac arrest
Ca	calcium; cancer; carcinoma
CAT	Children's Apperception Test
cath	catheter
CBC	complete blood count
CBD	common bile duct
CBS	chronic brain syndrome
CBV	central blood volume
CC	chief of current complaint
CCK	cholecytokinin
CDC	Center for Disease Control
CF	complement fixation
CGTT	cortisone glucose tolerance test
CHB	complete heart block
ChE	cholinesterase
CHF	congestive heart failure
CHO	carbohydrate
chr	chronic
CI	cardiac insufficiency
CIS	carcinoma in situ

Cl	chlorine
CN	cranial nerves
CNS	central nervous system
CO	carbon monoxide
CO_2	carbon dioxide
COD	cause of death
Compound E	cortisone
cong	congenital
conj	conjunctiva; conjunctivitis
CR	closed reduction
CrI to CrXII	cranial nerves
CRD	chronic respiratory or renal disease
CrP	creatine phosphate
CS	cesarean section
CSF	cerebrospinal fluid
C S resp	Cheyne-Stokes respiration
CV	cardiovascular
CVA	cardiovascular accident
CVC	central venous catheter
CVD	cardiovascular disease
CVP	central venous pressure
CVS	cardiovascular system
cytol	cytology
D	dorsal
D1 to D12	dorsal or thoracic vertebrae or nerves
DA	development age
D/A	date of accident or admission
DAP	direct agglutination pregnancy (test)

DBP	diastolic blood pressure
D&C	dilatation and currettage or currettement
DI	diabetes insipidus
dis	disease
disc	discontinue
DJD	degenerative joint disease
DM	diabetes mellitus
DNA	deoxyribonucleic acid
DNR	dorsal nerve root
DNS	deviated nasal septum
DOA	dead on arrival
DOE	dyspnea on exertion
DOS	day of surgery
D/S	dextrose in saline
DTR	deep tendon reflexes
DU	duodenal ulcer
DUB	dysfunctional uterine bleeding
Dx	diagnosis
EAC	external auditory canal
EBL	estimated blood loss
ECG; EKG	electrocardiogram
E coli	Escherichia coli
ECS	electroconvulsive shock
EDC	estimated date of confinement
EKG; ECG	electrocardiogram
EM	electron miscoscopy
EMB	eosin methylene blue
EMS	emergency medical service

ENT	ear, nose, and throat
eos	eosinophil
epis	episotomy
ER	emergency room
EST	electroshock therapy
etiol	etiology
ETOH	ethyl alcohol
ex	excision
exam	examine
F	Fahrenheit
FA	fluorescent antibody
FB	foreign body
FBS	fasting blood sugar
FDA	Food & Drug Administration
ff	force fluids
FH	family history
FHR	fetal heart rate
fib	fibrillation
FROM	full range of motion
FS	frozen section
FTSG	full thickness skin graft
FUO	fever of unknown or undetermined origin
Fx	fracture
g	gram(s)
GB	gallbladder
GC	gonococcus; gonococcal
glu	glucose
gr; grav	pregnant

MEDICAL ABBREVIATIONS AND SYMBOLS (CONT)

Grav I, Grav II 1 pregnancy, 2 pregnancies, etc.

GS	General Surgery
gt; gtt	drop; drops
GU	genitourinary
GYN; Gyn	gynecology
H	hydrogen
H20	water
HA	hemagglutinating antigens
HAI	hemagglutinating-inhibiting antibody
Hb; Hgb	hemoglobin
HBP	high blood pressure
Hct	hematocrit
HCVD	hypertensive cardiovascular disease
hd	at bedtime
HEENT	head, eyes, ears, nose, and throat
Hgb; Hb	hemoglobin
HGH	human (pituitary) growth hormone
HLH	Human lutenizing hormone
hn	tonight
H&P	history and physical
HPI	history of present illness
HR	heart rate
HVD	hypertensive vascular disease
Hx	history
IH	infectious hepatitis
IHD	ischemic heart disease
IM	intramuscular (injection)
I&O	intake and output

IOP	intraocular pressure
IQ	intelligence quotient
IV	intravenous (injection)
jej	jejunum
K	potassium
kg	kilogram
KUB	kidney, ureter, and bladder
K-wire	Kirshner wire
LBBB	left bundle branch block
LD	lethal dose
LH	luteinizing hormone
LOS	length of stay
LP	lumbar, puncture
L-S	lumbosacral
LTF	lipotrophic factor
Lues I, II, III	primary, secondary, tertiary syphilis
LV	left ventricular
LVN	Licensed Vocational Nurse
M	meter
M1 M2	mitral first, second sound
MB	methylene blue
MBP	mean blood pressure
MD	muscular dystrophy
MDR	minimum daily requirement
ME	middle ear
mg	milligram
m g	millimicrogram
MH	menstrual, marital, or military history

mHg	milliliters of mercury
MI	myocardial infarction
ml	milliliter
MMPI	Minnesota Multiphasic Personality Inventory
MR	metabolic rate
mr; mR	milloroentgen
MS	multiple sclerosis
MV	mitral valve
N	normal (concentration)
NA	Nursing Assistant
NaPent	sodium Pentothal
NB	newborn
NBS	normal bowel sounds
NC	noncontributory
N/C	no complaint
ND	normal delivery
NDF	no disease found
NE	norepinephrine
neg	negative
NIH	National Institutes of Health
NKA	no known allergies
NOR; Noradr	noradrenaline
NP	neuropsychiatric
NPH	no previous history
npo	nothing by mouth
NR	normal range
nr	not to be repeated
NS	nervous system

NSA	no significant abnormality
NSR	normal sinus rhythm
O	eye
OB	obstetrics
OBD	organic brain disease
OB-GYN	obstetrics and gynecology
OHD	organic heart disease
OL; OS	left eye
omn bih	every two hours
omn hor; oh	every hour
omn noct; on	every night
OPC	outpatient clinic
OPD	outpatient department
ophth	ophthalmology
OR	operating room
Orth	orthopedics
OS; OL	left eye
OT	occupational therapy
OU	each eye
P	phosphorus
P/3	proximal one-third (long bones)
p1, p2, etc.	para 1, para 2, etc.
PA	Physician's Assistant
P&A	percussion and auscultation
PAB, PABA	para-aminobenzoic acid
Pap test	Papanicolaou's test
Para	parous
path	pathology

PB-Fe	protein-bound iron
PBI	protein-bound iodine
pc	after meals
PCV	packed cell volume
PDA	patent ductus arteriosus
PDR	Physician's Desk Reference
PE	physical examination
Ped	pediatrics
PEG	pneumoencephalography
PGH	pituitary growth hormone
PH	past history
Phe	phenylalanine
phys	physical; physician
PI	present illness
PID	pelvic inflammatory disease
Pit	Pitocin
PKA	prokininogenase
PM	post mortem
PMH	past medical history
PMS	post-menopausal syndrome
PNa	plasma sodium
PO; postop	postoperative
po	by mouth; orally
PO2	oxygen tension
pos	positive
postop; PO	postoperative
PP	post partum
PPB	positive pressure breathing

pr	per rectum
prog	prognosis
ps	per second
psi	pounds per square inch
Psy	psychiatry; psychology
PT	physical therapy
pt	patient
PTA	prior to admission
PULHES	physical profile factors:
P-	physical capacity or stamina
U-	upper extremities
L-	lower extremities
H-	hearing and ears
E-	eyes
S-	psychiatric
PVC	premature ventricular contractions
PVD	peripheral vascular disease
pvt	private
qd	every day
qh	every hour
q2h, q3h, etc.	every 2 hours, every 3 hours, etc.
qid	four times a day
qn	every night
QNS	quantity not sufficient
qv	as much as you please
R	right
r	roentgen
RNA	ribosomal ribonucleic acid

MEDICAL ABBREVIATIONS AND SYMBOLS (CONT)

RA	rheumatoid arthritis
Ra	radium
RAIU	radioactive iodine uptake
RAP	right atrial pressure
RAS	reticular activating system
RBBB	right bundle branch block
RBC	red blood cells or corpuscles
RD	respiratory disease; retinal detachment
RDS	respiratory distress syndrome
rehab	rehabilitation
RES	reticuloendothelial system
RHD	rheumatic heart disease
RHF	right heart failure
RN	Registered Nurse
RNA	ribonucleic acid
RO	routine order
R/O	rule out
ROM	range of motion
ROS	review of systems
RR	recovery room
R&R	rate and rhythm
RT	reaction time
RTC	return to clinic
RUE	right upper extremity
RUQ	right upper quadrant
S	left
S-1 to S-5	sacral vertebrae or nerves
S-A; SA node	sino-atrial node

SAA	Stokes-Adams attacks
SB	stillborn
SBE	subacute bacterial endocarditis
SB test	Stanford-Binet test
SC	subcutaneous
SCD	service connected disability
SCM	sternocleidomastoid
SD	standard deviation
SDS	sudden death syndrome
SEM	standard error of the mean
SF	spinal fluid
sg	specific gravity
SH	serum hepatitis
SI	seriously ill
sib	sibling
SIW	self-inflicted wound
SM	systolic murmur
SMA	superior mesenteric artery
SN	student nurse
SNS	sympathetic nervous system
SO	salpingo-oophorectomy
SOAP	progress note format for POMR
S-	subjective
O-	objective
A-	assessment
P-	plans
SOB	shortness of breath
S-O-R	stimulus-organism-response

SQ	subcutaneous
staph	staphylococcus
stat	immediately and once only
STH	somatotropic (growth) hormone
Strep	streptococcus
STSG	split thickness skin graft
sup	superior
SVC	superior vena cava
sx	signs; symptoms
Sz	schizophrenia
T	Temperature
T&A	tonsillectomy and adenoidectomy
TAH	total abdominal hysterectomy
TB; TBC	tuberculosis
TBLC	term birth, living child
TBV	total blood volume
tds	to be taken 3 times a day
TFA	total fatty acids
TH	thyroid hormone
tid	three times a day
TL	tubal ligation
TM	tympanic membrane
TNTC	too numerous to count
TOA	tubo-ovarian abscess
TT	tetanus toxoid
TTH	thyrotropic hormone
U/3	upper third (long bones)
UA	urinalysis

UE	upper extremity
UGI	upper gastrointestinal
ULQ	upper left quadrant
unk	unknown
UQ	upper quadrant
UR	unconditioned response
URI	upper respiratory infection
urol	urology; urological
URQ	upper right quadrant
USPHS	United States Public Health Service
UTI	urinary tract infection
UV	ultraviolet
V	Volume
VA	Veterans Administration
vag	vaginal
VBP	venous blood pressure
VC	vital capacity
VD	venereal disease
VDG	venereal disease-gonorrhea
VDH; VHD	valvular disease of the heart
VIG	vaccinia immune serum globulin
vit	vitamin
VO	verbal order
VP	venous pressure
VPC	volume of packed red cells
VRI	viral or virus respiratory infection
VS	vital sign
WAIS	Wechsler adult intelligence scale

WB	whole blood
WBC	white blood cell
WCC	white cell count
wd	ward
WD/WN/BF	well-developed, well-nourished black female
WD/WN/BM	well-developed, well-nourished black male
WD/WN/WF	well-developed, well-nourished white female
WD/WN/WM	well-developed, well-nourished white male
WHO	World Health Organization
WIA	wounded in action
WISC	Wechsler Intelligence Scale for children (test)
wk	week
WNL	within normal limits
WR	Wassermann reaction
wt	weight
X	times
YOB	year of birth

MEDICAL ABBREVIATIONS AND SYMBOLS (CONT)

♀	female
♂	male
↑	increased; elevated
↓	decreased; depressed; lowered
↓↓	descended bilaterally
→	causes; transfer to
←	is due to
<	less than
>	more than
V	systolic blood pressure
Λ	diastolic blood pressure
O	absent; none
—	negative; absent
+	positive; present
⊙	start of operation (anesthesia record only)
⊗	end of operation (anesthesia record only)
	Upright. Vertical body position; body supported by lower extremities; torso upright
	Lying down. Horizontal body position
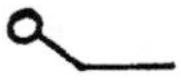	Leaning. Body trunk raised less than 90 degrees from primary supporting surface and supported by self or object.
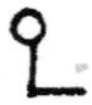	Sitting. Weight of body resting on lower part of trunk, back raised greater than or equal to 90 degrees.
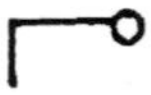	Leaning over. Dangling, any portion of body extended beyond the lower part of the trunk.
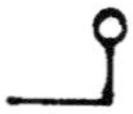	Kneeling. Supporting the body on the knees or legs.

1°	primary; first degree
2°	secondary; second degree
i ii iii iv v vi	amounts; dosages
Å	Angstrom unit
$\overline{aa}$	of each
$\bar{a}$	before
$\bar{c}$	with
Ⓜ	murmur
$\bar{p}$	after; following
$\bar{s}$	without
$\overline{ss}$	one-half
ʒ	dram; drachm
℥	ounce
fʒ; f℥	fluid dram; fluid ounce

COMMENT SHEET

SUBCOURSE MD0010 Basic Medical Terminology EDITION 100

Your comments about this subcourse are valuable and aid the writers in refining the subcourse and making it more usable. Please enter your comments in the space provided. ENCLOSE THIS FORM (OR A COPY) WITH YOUR ANSWER SHEET **ONLY** IF YOU HAVE COMMENTS ABOUT THIS SUBCOURSE..

FOR A WRITTEN REPLY, WRITE A SEPARATE LETTER AND INCLUDE SOCIAL SECURITY NUMBER, RETURN ADDRESS (and e-mail address, if possible), SUBCOURSE NUMBER AND EDITION, AND PARAGRAPH/EXERCISE/EXAMINATION ITEM NUMBER.

PLEASE COMPLETE THE FOLLOWING ITEMS:

(Use the reverse side of this sheet, if necessary.)

1. List any terms that were not defined properly.

____
____
____
____

2. List any errors.

<u>paragraph</u> <u>error</u> <u>correction</u>

____
____
____
____
____
____
____
____

3. List any suggestions you have to improve this subcourse.

____
____
____
____

4. Student Information (optional)

Name/Rank ____________________
SSN ____________________
Address ____________________
____
E-mail Address ____________________
Telephone number (DSN) ____________________
MOS/AOC ____________________

PRIVACY ACT STATEMENT (AUTHORITY: 10USC3012(B) AND (G))

PURPOSE: To provide Army Correspondence Course Program students a means to submit inquiries and comments.

USES: To locate and make necessary change to student records.

DISCLOSURE: **VOLUNTARY.** Failure to submit SSN will prevent subcourse authors at service school from accessing student records and responding to inquiries requiring such follow-ups.

U.S. ARMY MEDICAL DEPARTMENT CENTER AND SCHOOL Fort Sam Houston, Texas 78234-6130

Printed in Dunstable, United Kingdom

91220882R00125